DATE DUE

NOV 0 7 2007	
NOV 1 5 2011	

Baby at Risk

Baby at Risk

THE UNCERTAIN LEGACIES OF MEDICAL MIRACLES FOR BABIES, FAMILIES AND SOCIETY

Ruth Levy Guyer

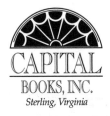

CAPITAL
BOOKS, INC.
Sterling, Virginia

Capital Books, Inc.
P.O. Box 605
Herndon, Virginia 20172-0605

ISBN 10: 1-933102-26-8 (alk. paper)
ISBN 13: 978-1-933102-26-9

Library of Congress Cataloging-in-Publication Data

Guyer, Ruth Levy.
  Baby at risk : the uncertain legacies of medical miracles for babies, families, and society / Ruth Levy Guyer.
      p. ; cm. — (A Capital currents book)
  Includes bibliographical references and index.
  ISBN-13: 978-1-933102-26-9 (alk. paper)
  ISBN-10: 1-933102-26-8 (alk. paper)
  1. Neonatal intensive care—Moral and ethical aspects. 2. Infants (Newborn)—Care—Moral and ethical aspects. 3. Infants (Newborn)—Diseases—Moral and ethical aspects.
4. Medical ethics. I. Title. II. Series.
  [DNLM: 1. Intensive Care, Neonatal—ethics. 2. Disabled Persons. 3. Infant, Newborn, Diseases. 4. Infant, Newborn. 5. Intensive Care Units, Neonatal—ethics. WS 421 G988b 2006]

  RG600.G89 2006
  174.2'989201—dc22

                                                                2006021841

Printed in the United States of America on acid-free paper that meets the American National Standards Institute Z39-48 Standard.

First Edition

10 9 8 7 6 5 4 3 2 1

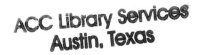

Dedication

To Mark, Anya, and Dana
With love and thanks for making my experience of being a mother
one that I wish every mother could have

and

To all of the parents who trusted me with their stories
and, of course, to their children

In memory of

Bill Silverman, pioneer and critic of the NICU,
who fought for justice for babies and their families

and

Brian Henry Schutzius, a lovely baby who was born at risk

Contents

Foreword

Ruth Levy Guyer's book is a meditation on suffering and hope, as well as a practical guide to the intricacies of the strange, fraught world of care for very sick newborns. No other dimension of the medical system involves so much weighty symbolism and grinding reality. No other population so challenges our capacity to cherish while exacting what could well be a thoroughgoing, lifetime commitment to a wholly vulnerable human being. No other kind of relationship than that with a gravely ill baby so tests our moral judgment or our ability to balance or to marry our interests with those of another.

Like Guyer, I have been awed at the strength of parents whose children have been born with severe impairments. Every time I visit a neonatal intensive care unit I feel embarrassment and shame at my petty concerns. At the same time the fact of these families raises profound moral dilemmas. How much can we ask of parents (admitting that they are nearly all willing to accept more than they would be asked to do)? How far must society go in rescuing those whose lives may include so little or limited human satisfaction (allowing for a wise reluctance to make a final determination about the "worth" of any child)? How careful should we be to alert prospective parents to the barely fathomable consequences of severe neonatal compromise (accepting that when new life is anticipated, denial may be impossible to overcome)?

The old saw that our technology has outrun our ethics has never been more true than in the case of imperiled newborns. Guyer's retelling of the history of newborn intensive care reveals not only a peculiar mix of compassion and voyeurism, but also how difficult it can be to perceive the harms that come with medical advances. Even now we are only learning the extent of the injuries that can accompany aggressive interventions on human beings who are at once so sick, so resilient, and so susceptible to long-term disabilities.

Guyer wisely avoids the armchair moralizing that so often accompanies discussions of neonatal illness. Staying painfully close to the ground with the families and children themselves, she sees the moral nuance that is too easy for distant critics to miss. Although our conversations about ethics often talk of choices, Guyer shows that such talk is far too static to capture the reality, when events and emotions overtake the protagonists. And yet, as she makes clear, to fail to try to anticipate the ordeal that may lie ahead is to fail to care.

Jonathan D. Moreno, PhD
Emily Davie and Joseph S. Kornfeld Professor
and Director,
Center for Biomedical Ethics,
University of Virginia

Preface

Babies are sweet, unselfconscious, and captivating. Like springtime, they represent hope and a fresh beginning.

Most are conceived easily, and most are born healthy. In fact, every second, forty-two new ones begin their lives on Earth. They grow, mature, and thrive.

But sometimes a baby is born sick or much too early. In the United States, for example, more than one in ten babies is born prematurely, one in one hundred is born with a congenital heart defect, one in five hundred has an X or Y chromosome anomaly, one in four thousand has DiGeorge syndrome (just one of many severe genetic anomalies), and on and on. At-risk babies have always been born, but such babies have not always stayed alive.

Technological developments in the last half of the twentieth century contributed significantly to the burgeoning populations of sick and premature newborns that we see today. Huge numbers of imperiled babies were born as a consequence of the widespread use of new assisted-reproduction technologies and in association with the highly risky pregnancies of older women and older men. New intensive care interventions were able to keep even critically ill babies alive. One medical team bragged that, with their technological expertise, they could "bring a peach back from death."[1]

These technologies did, of course, produce some spectacular and desired results—healthy babies or babies who were born sick or prematurely but grew into healthy children and healthy adults.

---

[1] Fred M. Frohock, *Special Care*, Chicago: University of Chicago Press, 1986.

But for millions of other babies, the high-tech interventions did not ensure good health or lives of high quality. Many babies born at risk remain trapped in lives that include profound pain, great disability, and little awareness of their environments; some lead lives largely defined by suffering. The parents, siblings, other family members, and friends suffer too.

I first began to see sick babies and talk to their stunned parents six years ago. How traumatic it was for these new mothers and fathers to give birth to a baby who might not live; how chilling to think that their baby might face a life of pain. The parents' plans and dreams were in disarray; their bewilderment was profound.

I was especially struck by how isolated each person I spoke with felt. They all described navigating through the world of sickness as though no one had ever traversed that territory before them.

I asked the families and myself some questions. What could be done to raise public awareness of the struggles of these babies and their parents? What should future parents know and what could they do to ease their own journeys through this world, should they find themselves there? Was it possible for some parents to avoid this world altogether? What about intensivists— doctors and nurses who specialize in intensive care: might they do some things differently? And how could individuals, communities, and policy makers help these families more?

The pain-filled lives of sick babies and their families raise so many knotty ethical questions. What is the purpose of a baby's suffering? Is it ever compassionate, kind, or fair to babies and their families to keep very sick newborns alive? Is it fair to the wider community to devote such massive resources to single individuals? Who should be speaking on behalf of a baby? Is it ever right for medical and nursing staff to act in opposition to the preferences of the baby's parents, when the parents are the ones who end up taking the baby home? Is it ever fair for parents or outsiders to insist that doctors and nurses provide care to babies whose situations are clearly medically futile? Why do we Westerners focus so much on mortality (death) but spend so little time talking about morbidity (suffering)? When is enough enough?

No easy or formulaic answers exist for any of these questions.

Parents, doctors, nurses, and others who are involved in a baby's care try to discern what is best for a baby and the family. Usually they are able to reach consensus at the cribside. But when there is a dispute, the parents or the caregivers can call for an ethics consult. Some hospitals have "beeper ethicists"; others have ethics committees. These people meet with the parents, the doctors, nurses, and other specialists involved with the baby to try to resolve contentious issues. The best or right solutions for each dilemma turn out to be different for each baby and each family.

When a sick baby is born, the family and the involved health workers are affected first and most. But eventually the lives of at-risk children affect the wider community, which may be asked to provide special education, special therapies, and special services for the child. Sometimes the responses of communities have been exemplary. But at other times, communities' responses and resources have been inadequate.

Sometimes legislators, public figures, and people who have no connections with and no responsibilities for a baby have imposed requirements on families and intensivists, almost always to the detriment of the babies. Babies, families, intensivists, and communities need better protection from the agendas of outsiders.

Decision making is never easy in emotionally charged settings. So many ethical dilemmas are laced with medical, social, economic, religious, and political issues, overtones, and consequences.

I was curious how the decision-making process actually takes place in neonatology, and so in the fall of 2000, I asked Dr. K.N. Siva Subramanian, the director of the neonatal intensive care unit (NICU) at Georgetown University Hospital, whether he would be willing to talk to me about decision making in the NICU. He said yes. For the next six months, Siva and I met regularly every few weeks for what were, for me, extraordinary conversations. Siva introduced me to issues, ideas, resources, and people, and we have continued these conversations—though not with such frequency—for the past six years.

The first families I interviewed were those whose healthy, thriving children were "graduates" of Siva's NICU. But Siva never pretended that every NICU rescue was perfect or even a success. At some point, he lent me a book written by Dr. William A. Silverman that described the dark side of NICU rescues. Siva said that he did not know the author personally, but that he did have his phone number.

I called Bill Silverman in late 2002 and set up an interview with him. Bill was in his mid-eighties at the time, a remarkable man still actively fighting for justice for preemies, blind babies, sick babies, and their families. As I describe in *Baby at Risk*, Bill was urging fellow neonatal intensivists to beware of the overzealous use of certain high technologies and to pay closer attention to what was happening to the children they were rescuing. Bill and I kept in touch regularly for the next three years. He sent me pre-publication copies of his editorials, and he directed me to new issues, new problems, and important stories in the news. My last email from him arrived just weeks before he died.

Bill connected me to other neonatal intensivists and to several parents. These people linked me to other individuals, to books, to documentaries, and to other resources. Through an entirely different pathway, I also started interviewing parents whose children were born with serious genetic anomalies.

Every baby's story is obviously much longer and more elaborate than the snapshot that I provide in *Baby at Risk*. Each story could fill its own book. The stories that I have included here are those of only about one-fourth of the families I interviewed.

Baby at Risk focuses on the personal lives of the babies and their families and does not describe how having a sick baby affected the parents' professional lives. Many parents whose children remain at risk and needy found that it was necessary to switch to more lucrative careers than the ones they had been engaged in; others stopped working altogether in order to provide full-time care for their child or children. Among the parents in these categories are a former opera singer, a Russia scholar, a lawyer, a member of the military, a social worker, a radio host, and a financial analyst, just to name a few. Not all perceived the shift to a new profession or to full-time childcare as bad, but it does give one pause.

Many families are stronger for their experiences. Many more, though, have broken apart from the unending pressures on them, and many of the parents have also had to cope with their own physical and psychological illnesses, which some believe may be directly traced to stress.

What I learned from my research is that keeping every baby alive but not really living has hurt many babies and their families, and this practice tends to devalue human dignity and personal autonomy. Medicines and technologies have no inherent worth; what matters is that they are used to bring about personal and social goods.

Westerners seem reluctant to engage in frank discussions about what interventions truly help babies and families and which ones cause more harms than goods. A commentator in one of the documentaries I describe in *Baby at Risk* (*When Miracle Baby Grows Up*) noted that any country that is rich enough to afford neonatal intensive care also has the moral obligation to accept responsibility for the care of impaired children throughout their lives, but that none of them does. It's time for this to happen.

I hope that *Baby at Risk* will help future parents learn more about options that exist for families of babies who are born imperiled. I hope that the exemplary neonatal intensivists I describe will serve as examples for their colleagues of what authentic caring is all about. I hope that policy makers will learn more about how to respond appropriately and proactively to the wide-ranging needs of sick babies and their families. I hope that the media will stop hyping "miracle baby" stories and start reporting truthfully about the benefits and the burdens of neonatal intensive care and new reproductive technologies. I hope that all of us can learn how to show more compassion toward babies and families, recognizing that the quality of a life matters and realizing that there but for fortune go you or I.

Ruth Levy Guyer, 2006

Acknowledgments

I have described in the preface of *Baby at Risk* how, six years ago, I began to think about babies who were born prematurely or gravely ill and about the ethical, medical, social, economic, religious, and political factors that affect and complicate their lives.

I am so grateful to Siva Subramanian, the director of the neonatal intensive care unit at Georgetown University Hospital, for introducing me to many of these issues and for discussing all of them with me. Siva's generosity to me has been unbounded—sharing with me his experiences, his insights, his concerns, his wisdom, and his time. He helped me sort through many of the complicated factors that affect the care of sick babies, and he never evaded a tough question that I asked him. Siva has described himself as an eternal optimist, and he is also a realist. He was the first person to tell me both heartening success stories from the NICU and also stories of how the NICU has failed. The first ten or fifteen interviews that I conducted for *Baby at Risk* were all with Siva. I don't think I have ever encountered anyone as universally loved, admired, and respected as is Siva. I witnessed his unstinting compassion for the babies in his care, their parents, and his co-workers and also learned about it from others. Siva is, in three words, the dream doctor. It's hard, even for someone who owns a thesaurus, to find enough superlatives to fully describe him, and so all I can do is thank Siva. I also want to thank Ninian Kring for scheduling my conversations with Siva and then rescheduling so many of them when the babies or parents required his attention.

I feel so fortunate to have known Bill Silverman. He was another doctor whose deep concern about and compassion for babies and parents was inspiring. Bill was one of the first doctors to work in a NICU, and he was also one of the first to recognize and worry about its dark side. He fought for decades to protect babies from unbridled experimentation in the NICU. Bill supported my research with ideas, contacts, insights, examples, anecdotes, and encouragement. He sent me a Ben Shahn portrait of Maimonides bearing the motto "Teach thy tongue to say I do not know and thou shalt progress." I treasure this advice from Bill, a courageous seeker of truth, human rights, and justice.

I am so grateful to Helen Harrison and Anita Catlin for many things—the interviews, of course, but also their willingness to suggest to me other parents and professionals I should meet, books I should read, documentaries I should watch, and so much more. Both also took the time to read this book in manuscript form and give me feedback. I am so admiring of the creative and innovative work that both Helen and Anita have done on behalf of babies and their families.

It is one thing to read stories of babies born at risk and something totally different to talk to the parents of these babies. I have been awestruck by the kindness and openness of the many parents I met and interviewed and so appreciate their willingness to trust me to retell their stories. I want to thank first those whose stories are included in *Baby at Risk*: Debby Barrett, Laura Fries, Wendy Greathouse, Gary Horn, Chris Keller, Alan Knapton, Diana Knapton, Lynn Kriss, Franky Lewis, Kathryn Neale Manalo, Becky Means, Mark Miller, Jack Schutzius, and the mother and father of the child I name "Graham" in the book. I know that for each parent reliving the experiences of their time in the NICU—even when the outcome was excellent—was extremely trying; I am deeply touched that they were willing to revisit those days. I know that these parents, especially the ones whose children are still at risk, have little or no discretionary time, and so I am doubly grateful that they gave me their time. They took a chance, and I hope that they are glad they did.

I also would like to thank the many other parents of sick and premature babies I interviewed whose names and stories do not appear in the book. They, too, were generous with their time and open and honest about their experiences. My conversations with them were crucial for assuring me that the stories I recount in *Baby at Risk* are truly representative.

I spent a wonderful day at the Georgetown NICU with Judy Diaz, who let me observe as she cared for three newborn babies. Judy also introduced me to many of the others on the NICU team that day. My earlier conversations with Judy were useful for helping me think about some of the factors that go into a nurse's perspective on caring for critically ill babies. It is easy to see why babies do well in Judy's care.

I want to thank Justice Maurice Amidei for discussing a troubling legal case with me and Brian Wallstin for sending me articles he wrote about the trial several years ago. Thanks also to Shari Finkelstein of CBS for sending me a copy of the *60 Minutes* episode that profiled the story.

I would like to thank Brian Carter for meeting with me to talk about palliative care and Andy Jameton for our discussions of justice and sustainability in healthcare. Edmund Pellegrino, Laurence McCullough, Susan Albersheim, George Little, and Jerold Lucey also were gracious about discussing with me various issues about the NICU; I am grateful for their insights and for their time.

It was such a thrill to chat with three graduates of the Georgetown NICU—Clara Knapton, Benny Kriss, and Meredith Kriss. Michael Kriss, the brother of the Kriss twins, talked to me about what it had been like for him—a six year old—to see his premature siblings for the first time. Thanks to these four for talking to me . . . and to the NICU for serving them so well.

During all of the years that I have been doing research for *Baby at Risk*, Martina Darragh at the National Reference Center for Bioethics Literature has, like a magician, made the most obscure references materialize. I thank Martina and also Dora Wong at the White Science Library of Haverford College for helping me locate the books and articles that I needed.

Students in my courses at Haverford College and Johns Hopkins University listened to some of the stories in this book and found them compelling. Their reactions and feedback convinced me that the stories are important, topical, and worth telling. I am grateful also to David Everett at Johns Hopkins for arranging for me to do a public reading of a section of the book when it was in its infancy. The response of the large audience that gathered that evening was extremely valuable.

My experience working with Capital Books has been ideal. Kathleen Hughes read my proposal, called me, and said, "I want to publish your book." She then made the process easy. She asked Amy Fries to edit the book and work with me. I cannot imagine having a more careful, supportive, or expert editor than Amy. Thank you both so much for everything that you have done to make this book come to be.

Chapter 1

The NICU Scene

Water began flowing from the faucets outside the neonatal intensive care unit as soon as the sensors detected our presence. Siva Subramanian, the director of the NICU, told me to scrub up for two minutes. I took off my watch, dropped it into my pocket, shoved back my sleeves, soaped my arms and hands, and stared at the clock.

Siva's two-minute scrub ended many seconds before mine did because he was in and out of the nursery all of the time and kept his shirtsleeves rolled always in the up position, streamlining his prep time.

Other sensors admitted us into the NICU. The overhead lighting was subdued. Rays of sunlight—reminders that there is a world outside—drifted in through a wall of curtained windows.

Most of the babies in the NICU that day were preemies, born weeks or months before they were due. A few others were full-term babies who were—or had been—critically ill. They, like the preemies, were in a struggle to begin their lives.

In the critical-care section of the nursery, all of the babies lay in clear Lucite cribs, tethered to monitors and bottles. Some cribs were aglow with a brilliant cobalt blue from bili lights that were helping the babies fight jaundice. A tiny boy tugged at the mask that was protecting his eyes. Several of the babies' heads were no larger than oranges. All of the babies had irresistible faces.

Next door, in the transitional step-down nursery where babies go to feed and grow, the scene was more varied. A baby was sleeping in a tick-tock swing, another was positioned upright in a molded red plastic seat, but most were just lying in their cribs, swaddled in classic, pastel baby blankets.

An alarm rang; a nurse adjusted a baby's breathing tube. Another nurse pricked a baby's heel and collected a sample of blood. As Siva and I walked along, a winsome baby girl who was not so heavily draped in medical paraphernalia idly raised her index finger, as if to signal hello.

Throughout the NICU, nurses weighed diapers and recorded the weights on charts. With so many babies around, I thought it odd that there was almost no crying. "It's hard to cry with a tube down your throat," Siva said.

There was no hubbub, no ER-style chaos. At least not then. But Siva told me that things could heat up at any moment should a baby become distressed.

NICU BABIES

People dream of having babies, but no one dreams of giving birth to a sick one. That's the turf of nightmares.

But here in the NICU, every baby was sick. Not one had been able to make the difficult transition from life inside its mother to living on its own. Everyone and everything in this wing of the hospital was focused on easing these vulnerable babies toward independent living.

Most of the parents would be taking a healthy baby home from the NICU. A tiny subset of these would be parents of the darlings of the media —the "miracle babies."

Other parents would go home empty-handed.

And still others would be taking home a child or children who had been saved but not "fixed." Some babies in this group would have minor problems. Others would be deeply damaged or debilitated by their incomplete development, their genes, a disease, the birth process, or the NICU interventions.

No one could know for sure which baby would have which fate, which one would end up doing well, and which one would not. Statistics never tell the future for any individual; they only summarize what happens to groups of babies.

As Siva put it: "We have no tools for prediction."

THE CENTRAL DILEMMA

Every medical intervention is risky. Each is essentially an experiment. And no treatment, however effective, succeeds for everyone who tries it. Even if a drug, a technology, a therapy, or a strategy works for 99.99 percent of babies, that still leaves the 0.01 percent group for whom the intervention will not be effective. With fifteen thousand babies born every hour of every day throughout the world and four million babies born each year in the United States alone, even excellent odds leave many babies—too many—sick with chronic problems.

In NICUs, for example, extremely immature and tiny preemies can be kept alive. Such babies are born long before their organs and systems are ready to work in air. Machines breathe for the babies' lungs and pump blood for their hearts. And while the machines serve as life-saving bridges for the babies, they sometimes also damage the babies' fragile lungs, fledgling blood vessels, and unfolding brains, often irreversibly.

NICUs are "horrible, wonderful places," wrote one physician/bioethicist. "They are the best and worst of pediatrics. They save many lives and they cause much pain and suffering. . . . The question that has hovered around these units since they were first developed in the late 1960s is whether we can have the good without the bad or, if not, whether the current balance of benefits to burdens is worth it."[1]

"If you draw a line," Siva said to me, as we talked about the dilemma of NICU rescues, "that is where progress stops. If you push the envelope, things might improve. But it's a catch-22. The question is, when do you keep pushing and when do you say 'enough is enough'?"

---

[1] John D. Lantos, "The Difficulty of Being Anti-NICU," *Literature and Medicine*, 1999, 18(2): 237–240.

Chapter 2

Born at Risk

CLARA

A prenatal test indicated that there was a hole in the baby girl's diaphragm. Her intestines had lodged in her chest cavity; they had squashed her lungs and had shoved her heart to the wrong side of her chest. The crowding in the baby's thorax had stunted the growth of her lungs.

The baby, who would be named Clara, was going to need surgery to repair her diaphragmatic hernia as soon as she was born. The surgeon would pull her intestines down and out of her chest cavity, reposition them in her abdomen, and then seal the hole.

The baby's parents, Diana and Alan Knapton, toured Siva's NICU at Georgetown University Hospital before Clara's birth because Clara would be recovering there.

"The hurricane was predicted for us ahead of time," Diana told me. She and Alan had not, like parents of preemies, been thrust without warning into the NICU. But then Alan turned to Diana and asked, "Do you actually remember *anything* we saw on the day we visited the NICU?"

Clara was born on January 15, 1995, and the corrective surgery went beautifully. In fact, the surgeon told Diana and Alan that it could not have gone better.

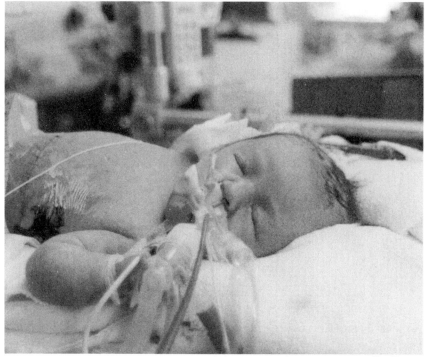

Alan Knapton

Clara at three days on a heart-lung machine

But later that night when Diana dialed T - I - N - Y—the extension for the NICU—Siva told her that Clara's heart and lungs were not working properly and not maintaining blood gases at appropriate levels. Clara would have to be placed on a heart-lung machine, which would supply oxygen to her blood and also pump the blood through her body. The hope was that her heart and lungs would then kick in and carry on for themselves.

Over the next few days, Clara was terribly, terribly sick. Her blood pressure was up and down; she received antibiotics, morphine, blood thinners. At one point she began to hemorrhage, and as blood poured into her tissues, she turned black and blue from her belly down through her legs.

Yet, despite countless setbacks, as the days went by, Clara seemed to be making real progress. One day, when her parents walked into the NICU, they saw X X X X X written across their baby's chest. The nurse responded immediately to their puzzled looks: she had not been playing tic-tac-toe on

Clara's body but was tracking her heart, which, amazingly enough, was migrating on its own across Clara's chest cavity to the left side.

On Clara's eighth day of life, she finally opened her eyes. At that moment, she fixed her attention on her parents and on the staff. And from then on, she stayed watchful and connected.

Fourteen days after Clara's birth, a young doctor in the NICU said something that frightened Diana and Alan. Babies on the heart-lung machine—it is called ECMO, for extracorporeal membrane oxygenation—must "fish or cut bait" by the end of the second week. If ECMO hadn't worked by then, it never would.

Another day passed, and then another, and another. On the nineteenth day, the staff slowed the ECMO pumps to see if Clara's heart and lungs could manage on their own. The attempt was unsuccessful. Alan feared that Clara might be one of the babies who had gotten "hooked on ECMO, with no chance of independent survival."

On the morning of the twentieth day, a brash young physician entered the NICU. It was now time, he said to Diana and Alan, to consider discontinuing support; the heroic measures had failed.

"Is this true?" Diana asked Clara's nurse. "Is there nothing else we can do?" Clara was so alert and so attentive. Her parents were sure she was improving.

The nurse agreed. She had a few ideas about other approaches that might work. By the next morning, new orders from Siva were in place giving Clara a weeklong reprieve. They would try to dry out the fluid in Clara's lungs and gradually slow down the ECMO flow.

When the day came to again try to wean Clara from ECMO, Diana and Alan woke up really fearful. But at the NICU, they found the mood to be electric. No one seemed worried at all.

And, it worked. Clara was successfully idled off ECMO and put on a high-frequency jet ventilator, which gave her hundreds of tiny puffs of oxygen each minute.

"When we saw her off ECMO and attached to the jet ventilator," Diana laughed, "she was vibrating a mile a minute."

Several days later, Clara actually extubated herself. Her wiggling and squirming had dislodged the breathing tube, but it didn't matter. She was breathing fine on her own. When Diana arrived at the hospital that morning, Clara was lying in her crib with her head sheathed by a foggy bell jar of

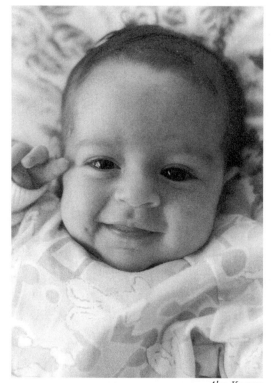

Alan Knapton

Clara at home and doing fine

oxygen. That was the first time that Diana actually saw her baby's "sweet rosebud lips." That was also the day that Diana felt she had won the lottery.

Clara soon moved to the step-down nursery and eventually went home.

Now she is just over eleven years old. She's an adorable, bright, sweet, spirited, and healthy girl, very artistic and charming and funny. She bears more surgical scars than most kids, but most of her scars are hidden, and they were clearly worth it. The bright eyes that her parents first saw on day eight are still probing, thoughtful, and expressive.

"I know that doctors have difficult decisions to make," Diana said, reflecting on their experience, now more than a decade in the past. "If we save this life, is it going to lead to more heartaches than anything else? I believe parents touch doctors emotionally. And I think that doctors get charged, like batteries, from the willingness of parents to fight for their children. The young doctor—the one who wanted to withdraw life support—seemed really humbled by what happened with Clara. And the surgeon told us that what Clara survived is nothing short of miraculous."

"Every baby is a miracle," Alan said, "but Clara is a double miracle."

DECISIONS

Siva said that Clara had truly been a trailblazer. Today, most babies who are placed on ECMO stay on ECMO no more than four days. Occasionally those with diaphragmatic hernias might spend as much time as Clara did on ECMO, or even more. But not back then.

And when Clara bumped up against the limits of his NICU's experience with ECMO, Siva had called around the country to see whether other neonatologists had discovered ways to improve ECMO's efficacy.

I asked Siva about the behavior of the young physician who thought the time had come to pull the plug.

"We do operate by paradigms for many situations, as that doctor tried to do," Siva said. "But all decision making is not medical. You have to make decisions on the basis of your knowledge at the moment and your understanding of the medical and moral dilemmas at hand.

"In addition to experience, information, and medical judgment, compassion is essential. There is *never* a precedent for a withdrawal of life support. I feel very strongly about this. A do-not-resuscitate order or an order to withdraw support from a baby should never become routine."

Siva said that members of the NICU team are not always of one mind about what can or should be done for a baby. They can disagree; sometimes they clash. The nurse knew more in this situation, and she intervened on Clara's behalf. This was, he said, a perfect illustration of "the nurses' intensity—working all day or all night long at the baby's side—and the physicians' intermittency."

DECISION MAKERS' DILEMMAS

"Any time a pregnancy ends with the birth of a sick child, like Clara, or with a premature birth, it's a shock," said Siva. "New parents whose babies are in the NICU try to face reality, but their reality is uncertainty. During the first days, everything is unreal. The parents go through all of the emotions associated with death and dying—denial, grief, anger, bargaining, and so on. For most, the experience represents a total loss of control.

"We have included parents in decision making for some time in our NICU. We say to them, 'This is your baby we are taking care of.' Most parents know that they are entitled to information and to participate in decision making. And they are very clear in understanding their right to express their autonomous choices."

Siva said his thinking about the central role of parents in decision making had been strongly influenced by one mother when he was a young neonatologist. He had connected her very premature baby girl to a ventilator. Within a few days of this birth, tests showed that the forced gases from the ventilator had destroyed most of the fragile blood vessels in the baby's brain. Her brain hemorrhage was bilateral, and it had the worst rating—grade IV. She would likely have profound disabilities.

Siva met with the baby's parents, a couple he characterized as earnest. He told them of the grim prognosis. The father wanted his daughter taken off the ventilator immediately. The mother hesitated; she needed more time to think.

Two days later the mother was ready to withdraw life support. By then, though, the baby was already able to breathe on her own. Siva told the parents that removing the breathing tube would not cause the baby's death. They wanted the tube removed anyway. The baby was extubated, and she continued to breathe.

Two years later, the mother burst into Siva's office, pushing her quadriplegic daughter in a stroller. She pointed an accusing finger at Siva and chided him for connecting a baby as premature as her daughter had been to a ventilator. "You were wrong from the start," she raged.

But how could he not offer the baby a 50 percent chance of a healthy life? Half of all babies attached to a ventilator would, according to the ventilator statistics at the time, grow up healthy, one quarter would die in the NICU, and the rest would, like this girl, experience bleeds and their debilitating sequelae.

"If one baby survives in this fashion," the mother had said, "it is not worth saving any of the others." She was angry and sad, she felt saddled, and the baby's father was long gone.

Siva had been thunderstruck by how passionately that mother spoke about forgoing opportunities for all of the other babies, the ones who could do well. "She gave me pause," he said. "She made me really think about a parent's perspective. I knew then that I couldn't make these decisions for families."

Then he recalled a second story from the same era, one that made him smile. A preemie boy entered the world at 28 weeks gestation, weighing just over two pounds. He was gravely ill and was put immediately on a ventilator. His diagnosis was respiratory distress syndrome; air was collecting in the baby's chest cavity—a condition called pneumothorax. He battled a variety of infections; at one point, he was suspected of having necrotizing enterocolitis, a condition that could destroy his gut. For some time, he could digest nothing. The complications mounted.

The baby's roller-coaster ride was rough and lasted many weeks. But eventually he grew strong enough to go home. The family moved abroad later in the year, and Siva lost contact with them.

Eighteen years later, the mother called to say that they were in the United States, and she would like to bring her son to see where he had been born. Could they meet with Siva? Into Siva's office strolled a six-foot-tall, handsome, strong, healthy young man just ready to start university studies at Cambridge.

"I've survived on that boost for years," Siva said.

Grave misfortune for one baby; an excellent outcome for another. And a crystal ball nowhere in sight.

Chapter 3

Birth of the NICU

BABIES ON THE MIDWAY

The impulse to save preemies and other so-called weaklings began in late nineteenth-century France, at a time when birth rates were plummeting. An obstetrician, Stephane Tarnier, saw a chicken incubator on display during a visit to the Paris Zoo. He was intrigued by the concept and immediately commissioned the manufacturer to develop something similar for the babies at the Paris Maternité Hospital where he worked. The quest to save French babies was on.

Soon, an obstetrician-inventor, Alexandre Lion, designed a more elaborate forced-air incubator, which he then took on the road. Lion exhibited his Kinderbrütenstalt—child hatchery—at the 1896 Berlin Exposition. And two years after that, an associate of Lion, Martin Couney, displayed French incubator babies at London's Victorian Era Exhibition.

The esteemed British medical journal *Lancet* enthusiastically endorsed the London show: "An extraordinary success . . . a serious exhibition where objects of art of great value were collected side by side with scientific inventions bearing on medical and public health questions."

But *Lancet* also noted that the exhibition was not "an unmixed blessing. It attracted the attention and cupidity of public showmen; and all sorts of persons . . . started to organise baby incubator shows just as they might have exhibited marionettes, fat women, or any sort of catch-penny monstrosity . . ."

The "serious matter of saving human life" was somehow getting mixed up with "the bearded woman, the dog-faced man, the elephants, the performing horses and pigs, and the clowns and the acrobats . . ." The babies at one exhibition, for example, were displayed opposite the leopards. Racing bicycles kicked up dust, visitors tracked in pathogens, and "the smoking of men" all compromised the health and environment of the babies.

The public, though, was captivated. People flocked to the baby exhibits. When the London show closed, Couney packed up his incubators and headed for the United States. He immediately set up the first of what would be his many American exhibits. By 1903, Couney was supervising a permanent installation at Coney Island that drew crowds from May through October for more than forty years.

A.J. Liebling profiled Couney in the *New Yorker* in June 1939. By that time, Couney's tally was 6,500 "saved" preemies. His empire at Coney Island had expanded to include two separate incubator installations and residences for himself, his daughter Hildegarde (a former preemie herself!), the head nurse Madame Recht, fifteen additional nurses, a chauffeur, a cook, and five wet nurses. Each wet nurse fed her own infant as well as a few preemies. And when she was not nursing anyone, she was expected to load up on milk-generating foods. "If Dr. Couney catches one have a hot dog or an orange drink outside," wrote Liebling, "he fires her."

Couney told Liebling that, when he gathered babies for the London exhibit from a French foundling hospital, the French gave him carte blanche: "*Prenez ce que vous voulez*," they told him, "take what you want." He bundled *les enfants* into three wicker baskets and headed for London. "Prematures, since they are almost insensible to their surroundings, have less trouble travelling than normal infants," wrote Liebling, and so "it is unnecessary to feed them during a journey of as much as twenty-four hours." For another European exhibit, Couney obtained babies from a German professor who "gladly loaned him six prematurely born infants from the maternity ward. This was considered a small risk, since they were expected to die in any case."

But when confronted with the accusation that he might be exploiting the babies by putting them on display and charging an entrance fee, Couney said,

"All my life I have been making propaganda for the proper care of preemies, who in other times were allowed to die. Everything I do is strict ethical."

Couney finally shut down his exhibits when Cornell's New York Hospital opened a special facility for premature babies. He is quoted as saying, "I made propaganda for the preemie. My work is done."

Bill Silverman, who was a pioneer in the United States in the care of premature and sick babies, characterized the period in which Couney was exhibiting incubator babies on the midway as an "odd chapter in medical history," yet one that was strangely contemporaneous.

"I find it hard to ignore the resemblance between the theatrics of the side-show exhibits and the dramatic actions in present day neonatal intensive care units," he wrote in 1979. "In both, I find a disturbing detachment from reality . . . The feeble infant is plucked up and deposited in a theatre-like setting in which superb technical experts make all-out efforts to support life. And when this had been accomplished successfully the infant graduates. But no comparable effort is mounted to deal with the enormous problems which face the graduate at home and in the community."[1]

DARK SIDE OF THE NICU

"The NICU in the United States today has gotten completely out of hand," Bill Silverman told me in 2002. "When I came into the field in the 1940s, the hospital environment for babies was simple—clean, warm. Nurses would feed the newborn babies. Those who were meant to survive did, and if they survived, they did well. Those who couldn't make it were allowed to die; they were said to be 'stillborn.'

"People in this country act as though there are no limits," he continued. "Yet there *is* a limit, because human reproduction is an imperfect process."

A human pregnancy should last forty weeks. But today, 12 percent of pregnancies in the United States do not. That translates to about one-half million babies beginning life prematurely each year in just the United States. In addition, many other babies remain in utero for forty weeks, as Clara did, but

---

[1] William A. Silverman, "Incubator-Baby Side Shows," *Pediatrics*, 1979, 64(2): 127-141.

are born with physical or functional anomalies because their genes, factors in their environments, or combinations of the two have upset their development.

Every newborn, whether healthy or sick, is unique. One nurse told me she considered all babies "designer babies," with their parts sometimes in novel locations or functioning idiosyncratically. Much about a newborn baby's physiology can be vague or unknown, and even unknowable.

Many interventions that save the lives of fragile babies are miraculous, producing immediate and obvious sought-after effects and solving the babies' problems permanently. Clara's experience is a good example of this.

Other interventions shore up babies through critical periods, but only as time goes by can the long-term consequences of these interventions—both the positive and the negative ones—be seen.

"I never wanted neonatology to be a specialty," Bill said, "because the focus is too narrow. It doesn't allow doctors to see what happens next to the children they save. It doesn't allow them to see the consequences of their interventions as they fulfill their personal rescue fantasies."

RESCUE FANTASIES

Bill had written a remarkable article in 1992—"Overtreatment of Neonates? A Personal Retrospective"—about his own freewheeling rescue fantasy.[2] The incident took place in 1945 when he was a young intensivist—a specialist in intensive care—at the Babies Hospital in New York City.

A baby girl—they called her Baby F—was born at 22 weeks gestation weighing one pound and five ounces. She was an "outborn baby," brought in from another hospital. Keeping her alive became what Bill called his "high adventure."

He pinned a how-to article that he found in the *American Journal of Diseases of Childhood* up next to the baby's incubator and carefully followed the instructions. He bolstered the baby's breathing with oxygen and monitored her temperature and eventually stabilized it. Twice daily he injected nu-

---

[2] William A. Silverman, "Overtreatment of Neonates? A Personal Retrospective," *Pediatrics*, 1992, 90(6): 971–976.

trients and fluids under her skin until she could be fed through a tube that was laced through her throat and into her stomach.

Then he began to improvise, going beyond the cookbook instructions. Each day he gave the baby small transfusions of his own blood—something that would be illegal today—on the chance that adult blood might have salutary effects.

The baby's parents were extremely wary, pressing him for assurances, which he knew he could not give, that his extraordinary efforts would result in a happy outcome.

Bill expressed hindsight horror at the "tunnel view" that had motivated him to sustain this baby's life irrespective of its possible quality and at his insensibility to the parents' personal and economic concerns. The parents were in their forties, and they already had grown children; the pregnancy had been a mistake, and they were very anxious about what the future might hold for this baby.

But at the time the rescue was taking place, Bill said he did not concern himself with whether he was doing what was right for the baby or her parents. He was bold, innovative, and he was showing himself to be a virtuoso technician. In fact, although Baby F died when she was three and one-half months old, she went on to hold the longevity record for more than fifteen years for babies born at the Babies Hospital with that birth weight.

Bill regretted that he had allowed his commitment to an "unshakable obligation to prolong life" to trump all other considerations. He had pursued his rescue fantasy while playing games with someone else's baby. Only later did he learn and come to appreciate that most "parents feared disability much more than death. They feared overtreatment and said so very directly," he wrote.

LOSSES FOR VICTORY BABIES

Baby F and other babies who were born in the United States at that time were called "Victory Babies." They came into a post-war world of magic-bullet antibiotics, Dr. Spock's just-published wisdom, and a national mood of optimism. State-of-the-art hospitals were springing up across the country. The United States was in love with technology, and anything and everything seemed possible.

The Babies Hospital opened a new, twenty-bed, premature infant station in 1949, and that's where Bill spent his time. Like similar units around the country, this proto-NICU was designed specifically for sick and tiny new-borns, and the centerpiece of its agenda was to reduce mortality among the low-birth-weight babies.

The premature infant stations featured cocoon-like, transparent incubators for the babies. Life-saving oxygen flowed into them, the air temperature was tightly controlled, and the babies were visible from every angle.

"Nurses and doctors stared at the naked babies as if they were seeing them for the first time," wrote Bill.[3] When the babies struggled and hungered for air, the staff cranked up the oxygen, the more the better.

But by the mid 1950s, some eight thousand "rescued" American babies who had started life small and sick were growing up blind. Stevie Wonder, born in 1950, was one of these babies. No one understood at first why this was happening, but eventually researchers connected the blindness—the retinopathy of prematurity—to the oxygen gas in the babies' incubators.

Studies in puppies, kittens, and other small animals showed that the growth of blood vessels is induced in the eyes of mammals during fetal development when low levels of oxygen bathe the peripheral retina. The incubator preemies—who, developmentally, were essentially still fetuses—were receiving massive doses of oxygen. Orderly blood vessel development around the eyes of the fetal infants was being stymied, and instead, the infants' vessels were forming in scattershot and chaotic fashion. Such eyes would never see clearly.

"I stare at the world through smeared and broken windowpanes," wrote one of the 1950s' incubator preemies in his memoir *Planet of the Blind*. "Ahead of me the shapes and colors suggest the sails of Tristan's ship or an elephant's ear floating in air, though in reality it is a middle-aged man in a London Fog raincoat that billows behind him in the April wind. . . . People shimmer like beehives . . . It's like living inside an immense abstract painting . . ."[4]

Bill noted that, although medical researchers were systematic and careful when they tested drugs and treatments on animals in their labs, "cautious rules were abandoned" when they faced all of the fragile preemies in the NICU. Some intensivists were thoughtful and hesitant—"let's wait and see"—but many had been reckless—"let's try it and see."

---

[3] William A. Silverman, *Retrolental Fibroplasia: A Modern Parable (Monographs in Neonatology)*, New York: Grune & Stratton, Inc., 1980.
[4] Stephen Kuusisto, *Planet of the Blind*, New York: Delta, 1998.

DESTRUCTIVE IMPERATIVES

The ventilators and other new technologies had dazzled and enticed the baby rescuers. They seemed to offer the solutions to the therapeutic imperative— Do Something! Anything!—of the desperate parents. The intensivists themselves often shared this desperation, searching fervently for ways to save the vulnerable babies in their care.

But while the ventilators were saving lives, they were blinding many of the survivors. And while they were sustaining bodies, their forced gases were shattering blood vessels and demolishing crucial structures in the babies' brains.

The ventilator quickly became the archetypal "halfway technology," getting babies only halfway to where they needed to be to lead healthy lives. They were among the first of a number of new iatrogenic agents of disease and injury—the medicines, the therapies, the doctors themselves, and the other interventions that hurt babies instead of healing them.

Bill grew increasingly uncomfortable with neonatology—with the technological imperative that was driving many intensivists to use new technologies simply because they existed even when they didn't make good sense, and with the team-think approach that was allowing individual intensivists to absolve themselves from personal responsibility for the pain and suffering that their interventions were causing for some babies.

(Team-think, he said, was Freeman Dyson's explanation for how the physicists who developed the atom bomb had been able to feel comfortable producing such a destructive device: "We did things together that none of us would think of doing alone," Dyson said. "Wherever one looks in the world of human organization, collective responsibility brings a lowering of moral standards.")

In the NICU, Bill said, the diffusion of responsibility allowed people not to worry about the "horrendous consequences of their acts."

Bill interviewed families of blind babies and rescued-but-sick ex-preemies and found that, while some parents were "ennobled," many were "boiling with anger" at what had happened to their children. Many complained of the "sacrifice test" they felt they were being forced to pass in life as they struggled to meet the needs of their profoundly disabled children.

Bill wrote of the chronic suffering and pain of so many NICU graduates and of the chronic sorrows of their families. He signed his columns and editorials and commentaries with his own name and also with the penname "Malcontent," and he wrote emails under the screen name "Fumer." He railed against the irrationality of many—though certainly not all—of the practices in contemporary NICUs and of the suspect entanglements of some NICU doctors with the financial successes of their NICUs.

Bill urged neonatologists to think more broadly and rationally and compassionately about what they were doing, about which of their ventures made good sense, and which were misguided and even self-serving adventures. He reminded his colleagues of the tragic lessons of the incubator oxygen. And he called again and again for more carefully controlled clinical trials in the NICU and for a halt to the epidemic of seat-of-the-pants experimentation with babies.

Parents whose babies were born prematurely in the seventies, eighties, and nineties and did not do well after their NICU rescues have often echoed his words.

Chapter 4

"Miracle" Mythology

DAVID

"My son David was 'created' by doctors," Gary Horn told me as we talked about the birth and life of his son David, who was born in 1993.

"Why did those doctors wreak havoc on this innocent child? They made errors of commission, not errors of omission. And although we are intelligent, the doctors treated us like children."

Gary's wife had just reached the halfway point in her pregnancy when she was admitted to a hospital near their home in Connecticut. She was bleeding heavily as the placenta began pulling away from the wall of her uterus. The doctors put her on bed rest to try to stanch the bleeding and control the abruption. But four weeks later, twin boys were born by Caesarean section.

The larger of the two fetal infants was handed to Gary by a doctor whom Gary characterized as the only compassionate one he encountered. Within an hour, the baby died in his father's arms. Gary said that he held the baby and he cried.

David was smaller than his twin. He weighed one pound and two ounces, but his lungs were further developed than were the lungs of his brother.

"I think that the NICU staff members went out of their way to hide information from us about the likelihood that David would have neurological

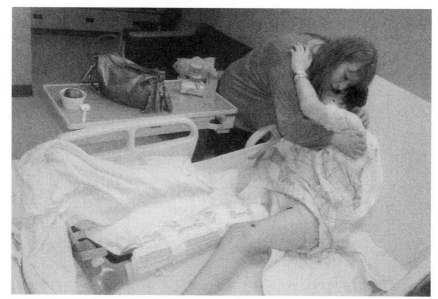

Gary Horn

David, at thirteen, and his mom after surgery to attempt to correct
"toe walking" associated with cerebral palsy

damage," Gary said. "I'm a math guy, and ninety-percent likelihood of damage is not good odds. If the doctors could not give David a reasonable chance
for a life of quality, they should have let him die. But the words 'quality of
life' never came up. The doctors were intervening, and the nurses at the hospital were complicit with them, saying things like, 'This baby is going to live!'

"The staff candy coated information or told us outright lies. We weren't
given guidance about, for example, what a grade III brain bleed was. They
said, 'He may be a little behind,' or 'Oh, well—sometimes these things work
out.' But they knew how paper thin the blood vessels are in the brain of a
baby that small."

David was thirteen years old when I talked with Gary. He was functioning at the level of a three-year-old.

"He has no friends," Gary said. "He watches Barney. His problems are
getting worse, but he's going to live. Who wants to have seizures? His life
sucks, and it adversely affects the lives of his sisters."

I was curious what Gary thought motivated the doctors to push so hard
to save such a young fetus. At 24 weeks, cells in the developing lungs are only

beginning to switch to a form that will allow them to facilitate the exchange of gases—a crucial requirement for living in air. And surfactant, the soapy substance that keeps lungs from staying collapsed at the end of each exhalation, is not yet being produced at all.

Gary mentioned several things.

"We had the bad luck of geography, being at a hospital where they save every fetus. And the doctor gave me some bull-crap line about Ronald Reagan and Baby Doe laws. But you know even small fish get thrown back.

"And there's the old story—follow the money. My insurance company paid $500,000 to this profit center. The doctors salvaged my son. They didn't save him. There are some things worse than death, and this is it. With David, my heart is broken every day."

MICHAEL

"If the doctors and nurses knew what our life was going to be like," Debby Barrett said when we spoke, "why shouldn't we have known? They need to be more honest with parents. Why did they tell me Michael would 'catch up' by age two? Why did we learn only when Michael was ten weeks old that he had retinopathy of prematurity? They had been checking his eyes all along and never even told us they were doing that. I only learned about it accidentally because I happened to be there during a handover. Why did they never mention that cerebral palsy is associated with prematurity?"

Debby had been admitted to a hospital near her home in England when this, her third pregnancy, was in its 20th week. She had been bleeding off and on for eight weeks.

Scans indicated that Debby had a complete placenta previa—the placenta was blocking the exit to her uterus. This meant that, when it was time for the baby to be born, he would need to be delivered by Caesarean section. For the time being, she was on bed rest and being observed.

At 2 p.m., five days into the 24th week of her pregnancy, Debby rang for a bedpan. As she was using it, the baby slipped out and landed head first in the cardboard receptacle.

She describes the scene and Michael's birth this way on her website: "The baby was curled up into a ball in the small end of the bedpan waving his arm;

he was still attached to the umbilical cord. For what seemed like an eternity, we all stood there staring at each other and at him. The midwives in there with me rang the emergency bell, and my little room looked like something out of Casualty. I've never seen so many doctors and nurses in one room. The umbilical cord was cut, the baby wrapped in a towel and whisked away."

Michael weighed one pound and fifteen ounces. He spent nine of the first twelve months of his life in the hospital, and his days there were fraught with interventions and crises—jaundice, bili-light treatments, blood transfusions, brain bleeds, retinopathy, ventilator support, lung damage, poisonous levels of blood gases, breathing and heart problems. At one point, doctors estimated that Michael's chance of survival was less than 1 percent. At another, his heart beat only four times in one minute.

"When Michael was just short of three weeks old," Debby said, "we had a discussion with the doctors about how things were not going well. I raised the issue of ending life support because I didn't want to see him suffer for the rest of his life, nor did we want to prolong the agony for him. The doctors told us they wanted to give him forty-eight hours more, he would be transferred from the ventilator to C-PAP [a different breathing device], and at that

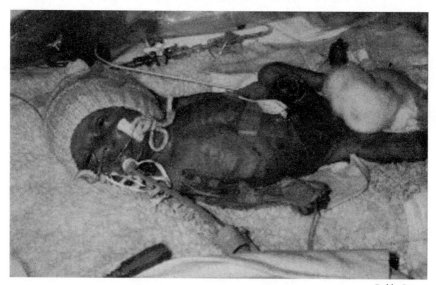

Debby Barrett

Michael at twenty days

point, a do-not-resuscitate order would be written. Martin and I loved Michael enough to be able to let him go, to prevent his suffering for the rest of his life. But we had never discussed that before with the doctors, and it was never mentioned again. I never felt that they listened to what I was saying."

No one listened; and no one talked to Debby and Martin about all of the problems that their baby was experiencing. One night, for example, when Michael was in the feeder-grower nursery, a student doctor came by and asked permission to listen to Michael's heart murmur. Debby said that Michael didn't have a heart murmur. But when the doctor confirmed that he did, Debby said, "You can imagine all hell let loose about how come everyone knew our baby had a heart murmur and no one had seen fit to let us know.

"We were so naïve. We thought it would be 'stick him in the incubator and he'll end up happy and normal.' When I went into hospital, I was told that the 'aim for' point for my pregnancy was 24 weeks. I was thinking that prematurity was like a bruise that would get better."

But Michael is now six years old, not toilet trained, and he will probably always need a feeding tube because he does not have a swallow reflex. He recently went back on oxygen at night. He has upcoming appointments with a cardiologist, a surgeon, and an ear, nose, and throat specialist, all to deal with acute problems.

Michael's medical chart includes a daunting list of labels: autism spectrum, hypermobility, learning disabilities, bulbar palsy, behavioral difficulties, severe speech and language disorders, attention and listening difficulties, chronic lung disease, intermittent oxygen dependency, retinopathy of prematurity, reflux, immunodeficiencies, and on and on. His sensory problems, combined with his lack of judgment, keep him constantly in peril.

"Michael can burn himself in hot water and not bat an eye," Debby said. He will put his face up close to an iron to feel the steam, and he will drag a chair over to the stove, climb up on it, and turn on all of the electric burners.

"I have to be honest and say I feel like we live in a prison," Debby said. "We're locked in the house because the outside world is not such a safe place for Michael, and yet neither is home. Everything has to be out of reach or locked away."

Windows stay closed, even in summertime, because Michael would think nothing of climbing out a window, no matter how high off the ground it is. The gate at the side of the house remains locked at all times, because otherwise

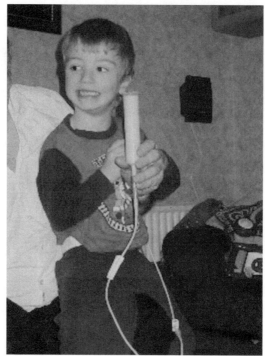

Debby Barrett

Michael holding his feeding tube

Michael would take off and disappear down the street. One day, for example, he slipped out through the gate, wandered down to the main road, and blithely got into a stranger's car. The driver happened to be a trustworthy person who went home and called the police to report that she had found a little boy.

"I feel I've been stuck on some kind of roller-coaster ride of ups and downs emotionally since the day Michael was born," Debby said. "I look back now and wonder how we are still in one piece. Lots of families aren't."

As Debby described more of the specifics of daily life with Michael, a picture emerged of a loose cannon racing around the house during all waking hours of the day. He "tears from activity to activity." He chews everything that he can put in his mouth—DVDs, jigsaw puzzle pieces, play-station games, books—although he doesn't actually swallow anything. He destroys the favorite items of his two brothers and his little sister.

"It has been heartbreaking to see things that we value and have worked hard to provide for the children be destroyed by a set of teeth," Debby said.

Michael's inability to swallow and his problem aspirating food into his lungs indicate brain-stem injury. Debby thought that it was equally plausible that his brain stem was damaged by the forced gases of the ventilator or by some mechanical injury (falling on his head into a sturdy bedpan?).

"If NICUs are to continue to save extremely premature babies, then the whole 'miracle baby' myth needs to be dispelled," Debby said. "People need to realize that these babies come at a price. No one warned us, for example, of the difficulties that kids with feeding tubes experience. We thought the tube would be in for a year and then be removed. But I've recently discovered that tube-fed kids don't stay dry at night, so the chance is that Michael will be in nappies at night for the rest of his life.

"If I remember the EPICure study correctly [a study of a group of very premature British babies]," Debby said, "forty percent of children who survived were left with long-term issues at age six. So there are at least forty percent of us with children who don't figure anywhere in the miracle world of premature babies."

"WHEN MIRACLE BABY GROWS UP"

In 2004, the British Broadcasting Company (BBC) aired a one-hour documentary—*When Miracle Baby Grows Up*—that presented the results of the study that Debby mentioned. The study was called EPICure—Extremely Preterm Infants Cure.

Researchers in Great Britain had been keeping track of every baby who was born there before the 26th week of gestation from March through December of 1995. Of the 4,004 babies born in that ten-month period, 1,200 were born alive, 811 were given intensive care, and 314 survived and eventually went home.

The study was sobering, an eye-opener for British neonatologists. They learned that the lives of too high a percentage of the survivors and their families were of low quality, painful, and joyless. Just doing "Something! Anything!"—responding with aggressive interventions to the therapeutic imperative—had not proved to be enough.

The program's narrator said that "by making this research public, doctors hope that in future, if parents ask them to do everything they can to save their baby, they will understand much more about what the future for that baby might involve."

Fifty percent of the children in the EPICure group were found to have disabilities by the time they reached two and one-half years old, and one-half of the disabilities were severe—blindness, deafness, cerebral palsy.

The 40 percent that Debby referred to was the percentage of children who had serious cognitive disabilities at age six. This contrasted starkly with the 2 percent of their full-term classmates who also had serious cognitive deficits.

The children in the EPICure study were nine years old when *When Miracle Baby Grows Up* aired, and by then 80 percent were dealing with physical or learning disabilities and impairments or both.

A pediatrician at Leeds University School of Medicine commented that "any country that is rich enough to afford neonatal intensive care . . . needs to understand that it also has a responsibility to those children as they get older if they are disabled, and we need to be providing them with the best possible care. Now, unfortunately, that doesn't happen. Once they go home from hospital they become Cinderella children."

He was not implying that the children were living with cruel stepmothers, but that the state had largely abandoned them and their families.

"Actually seeing the babies who come back with severe disability makes you realize that probably there is an outcome that is worse than death," he said.

"Intact survival may be a misleading term," he wrote in a medical journal that year, "as it is increasingly recognized that children who were thought to be normal, in the sense that they had no major neurodevelopmental disability at a young age, are now being shown to have cognitive, behavioral and dyspraxic [coordination] problems at school age and beyond. Although these may not be considered to be major problems, they do represent very considerable burdens of care and stress to the families and challenges to the provision of their education. . . . A surviving infant with multiple and severe neurodevelopmental disability may be viewed as a medical, social, and economic disaster."[1]

---

[1] Malcolm Levene, "Is Intensive Care for Very Immature Babies Justified?" *Acta Paediatrica*, 2004, 93:149–152.

The documentary also examined the more cautious practices and policies of the Dutch Pediatric Association, which, in 2002, stopped offering intensive care for fetal infants born at 23 and 24 weeks of gestation. Those born at 25 and 26 weeks were also no longer automatically treated aggressively. The Dutch physicians classified the older group as being in a "grey zone." Doctors would observe each infant in this group carefully before they would initiate any rescue efforts.

A professor of neonatal medicine at the University of Leiden commented that babies feel pain, that they don't have "a fun time" in the incubators, and that sometimes it was simply more compassionate to allow the baby to die.

"In the nursery we would be confronted every time with those very tiny, premature infants," he said. "They would do okay for a few days and then start to deteriorate and die. You see the pain of the child, you see the pain of the parents, and you start to wonder—are we doing the right stuff? For the baby? For the family?"

"Survival," he noted, "is clearly not the only, or, arguably, the most important measure of outcome."

Chapter 5

Comfort Care

OPTIONS

I had asked Bill Silverman what options existed for preemies and other critically ill babies besides the sorts of aggressive and invasive interventions that the EPICure babies, Gary's son, Debby's son, and so many other babies had received and were receiving.

Bill said that the most encouraging and compassionate option that he knew about for these early preemies and critically ill babies was called palliative care. He directed me to a protocol that Anita Catlin and Brian Carter had recently developed that explained how to provide comfort care to gravely ill babies. Bill was hoping that it might be more widely accepted and adopted.

"They take the baby out of the NICU," he said. "They allow the baby to die in a setting surrounded by family and friends. They stop the heroics; it's humane."

PALLIATIVE CARE INITIATIVE

In 1999, Anita Catlin, an ethicist and nurse practitioner, spent a year traveling in the United States talking to physicians and asking how they made decisions about resuscitating and treating marginally viable newborns. Of the fifty-four doctors she interviewed, not one had heard of palliative care, and not one had a well-formulated strategy for supporting a baby while the baby died.

Anita realized that textbooks and training manuals for physicians and nurses generally included chapters on bereavement, but that none of them included protocols for comforting babies and parents while the baby was dying. So ingrained in the cultures of both medicine and nursing was the equation birth = life that the possibility that a newborn might die instead of live was simply denied.

"Infants are not supposed to die," two physicians wrote not long ago. "They are the embodiment of new life and hope, which makes their death feel like a failure. Thus deciding to either stop aggressive therapies or withhold curative treatment goes against both our psychological instinct and medical training."[1]

Anita began to speak out about the dying of babies and about the fallacies of the technological imperative. She pointed out to groups of neonatal intensivists—doctors and nurses—that there were situations in which palliative care was wiser and more appropriate than aggressive interventions. She connected with pediatrician Brian Carter, and they then embarked on an eighteen-month project, along with one hundred advisors—physicians, nurses, parents, philosophers, administrators, hospice experts, pharmacists, funeral directors, and others—looking at how best to bring about more awareness among intensivists and parents regarding the possibility of offering dignified deaths for those babies who have marginal viability. This led to the publication in 2002 of the protocols for palliative care that Bill Silverman had admired.[2]

PALLIATIVE CARE IN THEORY

"The training of doctors is based on intervening to save life," Brian Carter told me as we talked in a coffee shop in Nashville, Tennessee, where he is a

---

[1] Stephen Leuthner and Robin Pierucci, "Experience with Neonatal Palliative Care Consultation at the Medical College of Wisconsin–Children's Hospital of Wisconsin," *Journal of Palliative Medicine*, 2001, 4(1): 39–46.

[2] Anita Catlin and Brian Carter, "Creation of a Neonatal End-of-Life Palliative Care Protocol," *Journal of Perinatolgy*, 2002, 22(3): 184–195.

pediatrician at Vanderbilt University Medical Center. "First you attempt to stabilize the patient's perturbed physiology; then you see the patient move toward health and the reestablishment of functioning, and maybe a cure.

"But with certain babies we may not be able to accomplish any of this. Sometimes it's simply not possible to ameliorate a symptom because the baby's underlying condition is too devastating. At that point, we have a professional responsibility to recommend a different approach—palliative care."

Brian had been struck during his training as a neonatologist by how inconsistent doctors' responses were when the babies they were treating could no longer be helped with technologies and medicines. Some of his teachers and colleagues had been proactive in offering dying babies comfort care, but others had avoided addressing the fact that the baby was dying. He had seen how their reticence needlessly stretched out the dying process, creating undue additional pain for the babies and their parents. This was what interested him in developing the protocol for palliative care.

He and Anita and the others on the project first defined the at-risk babies who could best be served by stopping interventions, and then they considered what approaches would make the end of life for the babies and their families easier.

Three general categories of babies, he said, were appropriate candidates for palliative care: the preemie who is born at the edge of viability and has very little chance to mature fully and develop properly and ever live a life of quality, the baby who is born with devastating genetic or physical anomalies for which currently there are no treatments, and the baby who has not responded to intensive care after a reasonable period of time.

"For preemies, biology is what really matters," Brian said, as he elaborated on the struggles of babies in the first category. "We dream that biology is less of an obstacle than it is. We think that skill and science are enough, but a baby's viability is absolutely contingent on biology. Even when two babies and two mothers are matched in terms of the mother's prenatal care, the circumstances of the birth itself, the baby's gestational age, and so on, it is the biology of the baby—can this baby's body respond to our interventions?—that either confirms or doesn't confirm that, yes, this is a viable baby. Sometimes the body works; sometimes it does not."

For the second group, the babies with severe genetic or physical anomalies, recommending palliative care is often harder.

"The baby may look well, yet it doesn't 'work' well," Brian said. "Sometimes people think that palliative care has an 'agenda' against disabilities, but that's just not true. It's important to parse the differences in disabilities and what we can do about them." Many genetic and physical anomalies result in low-quality or pain-filled lives, he added, but certainly not all of them.

In the third category are the babies who have spent months in the NICU but are not getting better. Brian described three babies who had been in the Vanderbilt NICU for five or six months each before a decision was made to switch them to palliative care. One baby had been born with severe physical anomalies—heart disease, organs outside the body; the second had an intestinal obstruction that burst in utero, and this had led to meconium peritonitis; and the third had a diaphragmatic hernia, but had not done well in the way that Clara had.

"For these three babies, intensive care was initiated at birth with all of the right intentions," Brian said. But each baby had gotten stuck: all remained critically ill, all had failed to make progress, all had stopped growing, and they were not likely to ever be weaned from the machines. Their problems could not be fixed or even managed.

"Every treatment is an intervention," Brian said, "but not every intervention is a treatment."

TREATMENT TRAIN

I asked Brian about the treatment train, which is a metaphor that is used to characterize how babies and caregivers get trapped in serial interventions. A first intervention, often connecting a baby to a ventilator, buys some time for a marginal baby and for the people who are trying to assess the baby and make treatment decisions. Often that is followed by a second intervention and then a third. Once a baby and the team get on this sort of train, it becomes difficult to get off.

"If you orient yourself strictly to cure and not to palliation," Brian said, "then usually what happens is you begin to face the baby's mortality too late. The train simply runs out of track; it screeches to a halt, or it runs into a brick wall. It's best once you are on the treatment train to make hourly whistle stops to reassess what's going on."

Something else happens when the treatment train is chugging along, accelerating, decelerating, traversing stable terrain and slippery slopes—the moral climate changes around the baby. Although medical ethicists say that there is no ethical distinction between stopping a medical treatment—withdrawing—and deciding not to start one in the first place—withholding—in practice doctors and nurses admit that they are loathe to stop a therapy once it has been started. So it is fairly easy to board the treatment train and extremely difficult to disembark.

If doctors can conceive of the train as one that makes whistle stops for reassessing the situation and reviewing possible outcomes, Brian said, then "eventually the treatment train concept may make palliative care work better."

PALLIATIVE CARE IN PRACTICE

Brian confirmed what Siva had told me, that it is never formulaic or routine for staff and parents to decide to let a baby die. But when all agree that palliative care is the compassionate and appropriate choice for a gravely ill baby, then the focus shifts away from the baby's medical condition and turns toward how to make the baby's remaining hours, days, or weeks of life comfortable and how to make this time meaningful for the family.

A photographer usually comes into the NICU to take pictures so that the parents will have a photographic record of their child's short life. Some NICUs assemble memory boxes for the parents that include clippings of the baby's hair, footprints or handprints, name bands, crib cards, and other mementos.

Brian recalled that the parents of one baby in his NICU organized a party outside in the sunshine for the staff, the family, and the baby. After the gathering—a celebration of the baby's short, difficult life—the family left the NICU and moved into a private room, where the baby could die.

Brian said that the decision to switch a baby to palliative care can have profound effects, not just on the family and the baby, but also on the NICU staff. Neonatal intensivists care deeply about the babies in their care; they also can anguish over providing care that they feel is ineffectual, inappropriate, futile, or painful for a baby. Providing palliative care to a struggling baby can thus be therapeutic for intensivists, reducing some of their well-known occupational hazards—stress, burnout, compassion fatigue, and depression.

(One nurse I spoke to said that the babies she remembers most are "those I help go. This is where, as a nurse, I am really critical.")

"Sometimes we feel the toll of six deaths in a week," Brian said, "and of course there is a lot of drama around a six-month hospitalization. These things affect us . . . and they should."

TABOO SUBJECT

The wrenching decisions to allow a baby to die and to actively ease the baby's death with palliative care are probably made much harder than they need to be for intensivists and parents in the United States because a thick shroud of silence hangs over the subject of infant mortality. But between twenty-five thousand and thirty thousand U.S. infants die each year before they have reached their first birthdays. If most of these deaths are inevitable, why aren't they discussed?

Why is there not more open and honest discourse about life's limits (even at the beginning of life), about the limits of technologies, and about the fact that not every baby fares well, even after aggressive interventions?

Why also do we spend so little time discussing and addressing morbidity—the lifelong suffering—that comes when aggressive intensive care has failed to *fully* rescue a baby?

Can the myth of the "miracle baby" be dispelled, as Debby suggested?

When will the media stop hyping stories of the "miraculous" births of septuplets and other higher multiples and instead report on how many of the infants go home with severe disabilities or never actually go home at all?

What if the topic of infant death were not taboo? Parents and intensivists could grieve more openly, and they might receive better emotional support from others in the community. They would not be left feeling that their personal failures were responsible for the baby's death. Dying babies would receive more timely comfort care, they would be subjected to fewer pointless and painful interventions, and they could then die more peacefully.

DYING WITH DIGNITY

A moving memoir by Amy Kuebelbeck, *Waiting for Gabriel,* describes how one family deliberated and eventually chose palliative care for their son.[3] She and her husband were forewarned by a prenatal test that their baby would be born with hypoplastic left heart syndrome, a condition for which a series of risky heart surgeries over several years could still not assure the baby of a healthy life. They concluded, months before Gabriel's birth, that they were not going to give him anything but comfort care when he was born.

Because the Kuebelbecks were able to think through how to make Gabriel's short life soothing for him and meaningful for themselves—he died two hours and twenty-eight minutes after he was born—their baby's death was dignified. As the parents wrote on the announcements that they sent out, Gabriel was

> *Perfect except for his heart.*
> *Died peacefully in our arms.*
> *Surrounded by people who love him.*
> *He knew only love.*

Amy Kuebelbeck acknowledged that circumstances would be different for each family and that the choice that each family makes is intensely personal. She understood that what was right for her family might not be right for others.

"No part of our story is meant to criticize the decisions of parents who pursue medical treatment for their beloved little ones," she wrote. "All of us had to sort through conflicting medical opinions, and all of us made our decisions with love for our babies foremost. . . . What parents want to bury their baby? Indeed, we might have turned to surgery too if we had learned of Gabriel's heart after he was born and had to make a decision immediately, in a state of shock. We too might have pleaded with the doctors, 'Do anything! Just save our baby.'"

"When doctors don't recommend palliative care," Brian Carter said to me, "it may be because they have not yet reconciled a peace with life being finite. If they don't feel comfortable about their own mortality, they may not feel comfortable with the dying of their patients."

---

[3] Amy Kuebelbeck, *Waiting for Gabriel*, Chicago: Loyola Press, 2003.

Chapter 6

Parents Matter

DECISION MAKERS

"First, Do No Harm" and its corollary "Do Good" are two of the fundamental dictums of medicine. All doctors swear to uphold these key principles, which are known in the vernacular of medical ethics as nonmaleficence and beneficence.

We like to think that all doctors are beneficent, nonmaleficent, and act fully professionally at all times. Realistically, we also know that personalities and personal beliefs differ and that beliefs influence and drive actions and behavior.

Doctors, like parents, do not all share a single perception of what it means to do good and to do no harm, and any two doctors' definitions of what is good for a baby—what is in the baby's best interests—and also what is in the best interests of the baby's family may be quite discrepant. Thus, decisions that are made regarding actions to take on behalf of a baby and what actually happens to a baby in the NICU can range enormously, depending on who is taking care of the baby.

Before healthcare became a big business and, as is so common today, an impersonal enterprise, most people knew their doctors well. They trusted their chosen physicians and generally deferred to their expert medical opinions. Doctors usually acted paternalistically, and patients were comfortable with that; and both parties accepted that the doctor would serve as the medical decision maker and watchful shepherd for the vulnerable patient.

But in the 1960s, around the time that NICUs were beginning to assume their current high-tech configurations, various rights movements—civil rights, women's rights—and, later, the patients' rights movement helped parents understand the concepts of empowerment and autonomy. Parents then began to challenge physician paternalism and the standard structure of the physician-patient relationship.

Parents appreciated that more than one point of view might be valid when it came to medical interventions, especially in situations of great uncertainty. They realized that they could make sensible decisions for their babies without having any special medical or nursing expertise because the dilemmas they faced in the NICU often entwined ethical with medical choices. A push began for more autonomy for parents, particularly in the community of parents of marginally viable micropreemies—those babies born at extremely low birth weights.

Frequently, a productive collaboration would ensue. Many doctors saw that shared decision making with a baby's parents was an enlightened approach for coping with the uncertain outcomes that characterized the world of neonatology, and they felt comfortable working in partnership with the baby's parents. Shared decision making generally left parents feeling better satisfied with the outcome, no matter what it was. As Siva, Bill, and Brian all said to me repeatedly, the values of the parents and the social and religious and cultural circumstances of the family really mattered. Babies were not on their own—they existed in the contexts of their families.

But sometimes what happened in the NICU was not collaboration but collision. Some doctors were loathe to give up their positions as the primary decision makers, and even today some continue to cling to the old paternalism.

In situations where the baby has done well despite a cribside battle over autonomy, the parents may quickly be able to forget that their preferences were ignored.

But when a child goes on to lead a difficult life—one of enduring pain, constant suffering, great disabilities—then the parents may continue to ask, and justifiably, how it is that none of the doctors who were dismissive of their preferences or the institutions that imposed these aggressive overtreatments on their child end up bearing any lasting responsibilities for the lifelong care of the child.

KEEGAN AND HOLLY

"The joy and miracle of having a baby is, for some families, short lived," the narrator said on New Zealand's TV 3 in July 2005. Thus began the segment "Miracle Babies" on New Zealand's *60 Minutes* show.

The program was focusing on two prematurely born children—Keegan Lewis and Holly Ross—and their parents Franky and Tony Lewis and Leesa and Lance Ross.

Leesa talked about her shock upon first seeing her baby Holly. "She looked awful. I didn't think she was a miracle baby."

Yet a doctor in the hospital had dismissed the obvious crisis with a commonplace simile—he explained to Leesa and Lance that the baby, like a half-cooked chicken, would in time "be done."

But there had been no cooking-to-completion for Holly in the NICU, or afterward, just suffering for the baby and her parents.

"All she did was scream," Leesa said. "I never thought a baby could scream that much."

The camera zoomed in on Holly, who was eight years old. She could not speak, but she had just learned how to give a kiss, a winning move that most healthy infants master in their first months of life.

The cameras panned to Keegan, who had just turned nine years old. Four people hoisted his limp, rag doll's body onto a horse so that he could ride the horse around a ring. Later, the cameras showed Keegan in his wheelchair, grinning and singing in the school assembly.

Keegan, too, had cried continuously as an infant, his parents said. And the relentless crying of both children had been devastating for all four parents to watch and exhausting for them to endure.

"I love her dearly," Leesa said. "She works really hard. But she is really hard work. She's trapped in that horrible body."

The narrator noted that both families were doing everything in their power to give their children's lives "quality," but that it was extremely difficult to do this for children with such profound disabilities without adequate support.

The host wrapped up the segment with the observation that "both families are waiting for a miracle."

Franky, Tony, Leesa, and Lance had reached their breaking points. They had not just been caring around the clock for their profoundly disabled children, but they also had been battling the health authorities for every service, every piece of equipment, and everything else that their children needed. Their lives did not seem to reflect what the New Zealand Ministry of Health had announced in 2001 as its official Disability Strategy—to make life better, through inclusion, for citizens who had long-term disabilities and for their families.

"The Disability Strategy says that families need to be valued," Franky Lewis explained to me over the telephone. "I didn't feel valued. So I thought: what am I going to do about it?"

At first Franky wrote letters to the Health Ministers.

"These people are elected by us, and if we don't let them know what's happening, nothing is going to change," she said. "I realized that the Ministry of Health had no clue what a day in our life is like. I thought if we could be proactive ourselves, that's the best way to raise awareness. If you are cool headed, peaceful, going for a goal, and if you don't let your emotions out, you can plant little seeds for change. But when you *whinge*, people go into defensive mode."

Franky's requests elicited written responses from the Ministers, but not much was changing. So in frustration, she and Tony and the Rosses decided to go public.

They posted a short document on the Internet—*Miracle Babies Grow Up With Problems* (http://www.proactiveparents.co.nz/about.htm).

"Within an hour of posting our document," Franky said, "we had *60 Minutes* knocking at our door."

The web document is straightforward. On the opening page, the families introduce themselves.

"We are two families affected by the very high needs of our children . . . We have reached the point where we just cannot go on anymore. We are physically, mentally, emotionally and financially strained and are left with no option but to try to gain acknowledgement of our situation in order to be able to live decent and meaningful lives and secure our children's futures in terms of adequate support."

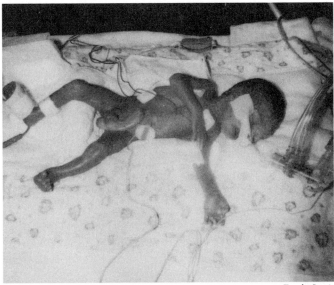

Franky Lewis

The first picture of Keegan

The next page presents a short profile of Keegan, who was born in 1996 at 26 weeks gestation weighing one pound twelve ounces. Doctors had jumped in and resuscitated him—he was not breathing—without consulting Franky and Tony. Keegan stayed in the NICU for three months and then went home. But back at home, his parents faced continuing stresses: diagnoses—cerebral palsy, epilepsy—hernia surgeries, "autistic" behaviors and cognitive difficulties, and "a long learning curve" of other challenges. The assurance they were given by the pediatric consultant at the hospital that the National Health system would cover everything Keegan needed proved completely untrue. Franky and Tony were fighting the National Health constantly just to meet Keegan's daily needs.

The next web page profiles Holly, who was born in 1997 at 27 weeks. She weighed two pounds, and her parents characterized her birth as "horrific"— an emergency Caesarean section that left her bruised and even lacerated. Holly, like Keegan, was not breathing at birth, was resuscitated—also without a consultation with the parents—and given a blood transfusion. When Holly went home at three months, she had significant breathing, respiratory, and motor problems, and brain damage.

After that, they list the children's unofficial labels—autism, Asperger's, global delay, dyslexia, dyspraxia, attention deficit disorder, and so on. Neither sleeps; both are high functioning and intelligent but unable to interact and connect with their environments; both are regularly frustrated and often sick.

The children both endure "endless medical interventions and their little bodies suffer continuous and tremendous physical pain," wrote the parents. "They live in a different world, don't adapt easily to ours, and being the buffer between their world and the outside world is a very challenging task. . . . And what makes it hard to get on with is that our society doesn't acknowledge their very high needs. We . . . provide 24-hour specialised care . . . [and] spend the equivalent of a full-time job fighting for our children's needs . . . If funding keeps being 'rationed,' we will have to declare ourselves unfit and unequipped to look after our own children . . . We do not want to give up on our children. Our children deserve and have the right to enjoy all the experiences of being part of a family . . . However, to do this, families [need] sufficient support."

The posting ends with a list of what the couples want: public acknowledgment of their situations, the equipment their children need, an end to the bureaucratic waiting lists, support at home and in school, and respite help. They want the Ministry of Health to treat them fairly and proactively. And they wrote, "We would like scientists to stop playing God with other people's lives."

The *60 Minutes* segment elicited emails from many parents whose children were similarly disabled, as well as offers from people who wanted to help out financially. The two couples were excited about the prospect of collaborating with a group of families who could work together to lobby for services and inclusion.

"We feel that making a lot of noise is the only way to be heard and to get the Ministry of Health to let us take a proactive role in deciding how to meet the needs of our disabled families," they wrote in their November 2005 update.

"We need to make decisions as a society," Franky told me. "If a baby is born and needs extensive care to survive, is all of that going to lead to a dignified life? I'm still thinking about these issues. Wouldn't it be more peaceful to learn from a death instead of trying to preserve life at all cost? Keegan, for example, has a rough life. He deals daily with the consequences of prematurity. He has impaired cognition, he needs constant reassurance, he needs to

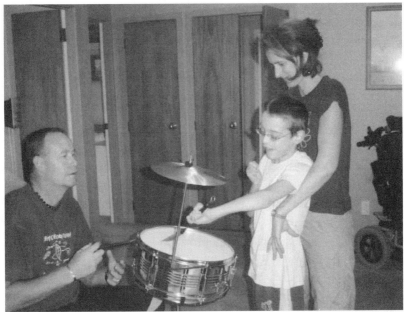

Franky Lewis

Keegan playing drums with his parents' help

learn how to do everything, and it takes a very long time for him to learn each thing. For example, he struggles daily with mind-body awareness. I do yoga with him; it's helping him physically, it's calming, and it is improving his awareness. But he constantly needs to know whether he is well or sick.

"If we'd been given the choice, we might not have resuscitated Keegan. But it is really hard to go back in time to think what I would have done 'if.' If you see the doctor trying to resuscitate your baby, you think, 'I hope he's not going to die.' You don't have time to think 'is that the best for our family?'

"You have to take charge of your life; you can't just rely on others to change it. I just made an appointment with the National Manager for Disability Support Services to spend a full day with us during next school holidays to see what our life is like.

"I believe in concentrating on the positive—like discovering and seeing the beauty in my child's eyes. How else could I raise him to become balanced and happy?

"We also need to plant seeds to change things, to raise awareness. Neonatologists have no idea what sorts of disabilities our kids are growing up with, and they don't always know what they are doing. We need to make contact with them to tell them what it is like for us, to keep raising their awareness."

PARENTAL ACTIVISM

"It's just cruel to put families and babies in situations where the outcomes are so bad," Helen Harrison said as we talked in the lobby of the Omni Hotel in Washington, D.C. She was attending the 2005 Hot Topics in Neonatology meeting, which brings neonatal intensivists together from all over the world to discuss innovative and controversial treatments for newborns.

Helen, unlike most of the other 1,450 participants at the meeting, had not actively chosen neonatology as a profession. She had been thrust unexpectedly into the field in 1975, when her first baby was born prematurely at 29 weeks gestation.

Helen's son Edward weighed two pounds and thirteen ounces at birth. He was bruised from his rapid birth and covered in a pinpoint rash from the lis-

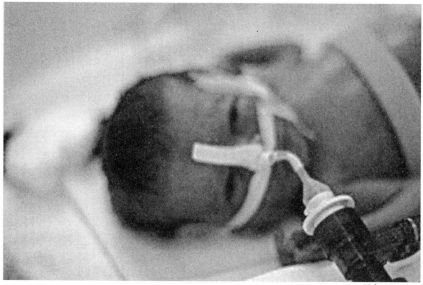

Helen Harrison

Edward connected to a respirator

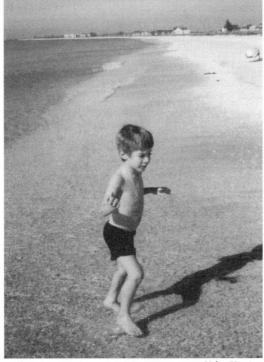

Helen Harrison

Edward at age six

teria infection that had triggered Helen's early labor. He was not expected to survive—"Don't even hope," said the neonatologist—but Edward did survive.

Then, during Edward's first week of life, he suffered a massive brain hemorrhage. Everyone agreed that the respirator should be turned off. As one of the doctors put it, "We don't think he has enough brain left ever to breathe on his own."

But Edward managed to breathe on his own. And he weathered what Helen termed myriad cataclysmic events around his birth. Against all odds, Edward remained alive.

Helen's response to the premature birth and to life with a profoundly disabled and needy baby was proverbial—lemons to lemonade. She researched infant development, prematurity, and NICU procedures, and she solicited stories from other parents. When Edward was eight, she published *The Premature*

Baby Book, a comprehensive account of prematurity, experiences of parents and babies, practical advice, resources for parents and disabled children, guidelines for navigating the world of the sick, and basic information about the medical and social realities of being the parent of a preemie.

The Premature Baby Book drew other parents to Helen. Over the years, she and the others formed networks—first locally and then, of course, globally, thanks to the Internet. And today she remains one of the most vocal and visible parent advocates for justice for preemies and their parents in the United States.

PRINCIPLES FOR FAMILY-CENTERED CARE

Helen began attending Hot Topics meetings in 1992 at the invitation of Jerold Lucey, the chairperson of the conference and longtime editor of the medical journal *Pediatrics*. She and ten other parents had been working with Lucey and a group of doctors that year to draft guidelines for improving the NICU experiences of parents and at-risk babies. The collaboration came about at Lucey's suggestion, after Helen had forwarded letters to him from disgruntled parents who had written to her about their traumatic NICU experiences.

The parent-physician group met for three days in Burlington, Vermont, that June. The document that they produced—"The Principles for Family-Centered Neonatal Care" ("The Principles")—outlined ways to empower parents, to improve communications between parents and intensivists in the NICU, and to protect babies from unnecessary, painful, and experimental procedures. "The Principles" was published in *Pediatrics* in November 1993.

The document is practical. It calls for frank and open discussions between parents and intensivists about various interventions and their likely risks, benefits, and outcomes. It recommends ongoing conversations about the baby's medical condition and also what might be the related ethical and social implications of certain interventions.

To facilitate communication and understanding, "The Principles" suggests that parents be given complete access to the baby's chart—including writing their own version of the baby's "story" on the chart—and that parents be included in rounds at which their baby is discussed.

"The Principles" also calls for better management of pain. Odd as it seems, babies were long considered to feel no pain. But anyone close to a baby can easily recognize the great capacity of babies to suffer. "The Principles" lists many of the obvious triggers of pain for babies in the NICU—needle sticks, breathing tubes, surgery, other invasive procedures—as well as less obvious secondary sources that also could harm babies—noise, bright lights, bustle, and other disturbances of the environment. (The pain of infants is now universally acknowledged; researchers have identified some biochemical markers of pain, and these markers can be closely monitored. And many of the environmental sources of pain have been remediated.)

"The Principles" asks that all new treatments be introduced only in the context of properly controlled clinical trials. Intensivists are urged to be completely transparent as they explain to parents which interventions have been well vetted in clinical trials and are reliably safe and which ones are still in experimental stages. As for impromptu seat-of-the-pants experiments, "The Principles" makes no provision for them.

Finally, "The Principles" calls for more training for parents in how to manage their at-risk babies at home and for more exposure of intensivists to NICU graduates as the babies grow up. Such follow-up studies would, as Bill Silverman had urged, help intensivists appreciate what happens to the babies they save.

The parents who helped draft "The Principles" understood that their own children—twenty preemies, many of whom were growing up with profound physical, cognitive, and medical problems—would not benefit from the proposed changes. Their work was altruistic, done for the benefit of future babies and their parents.

COLLIDING WORLDS: REAL AND IDEAL

In an ideal world, every intensivist in every NICU would have understood the value of "The Principles" and would have adopted the recommendations, and all parents of NICU babies would read and understand their rights and responsibilities.

In such a world, all parents would today be leaving the NICU satisfied that their preferences had been acknowledged and honored. All babies would be benefiting from the double protection of informed parents and caring intensivists, and they would be spared from inappropriate overtreatments and from being unwitting targets of "unthinking medical activism."

But while the interpersonal climate has improved in most NICUs—with more dialogue and more democratic decision making going on—babies still at times receive aggressive and inappropriate interventions now, more than a decade after "The Principles" was published.

Often intensivists are still at fault. But not always.

Sometimes parents push too hard for treatments that are medically inappropriate. Some of these individuals relied on reproductive technologies in order to conceive a baby and then expect that other technologies will rescue and maintain their baby.

Some parents are simply uninformed or ill informed, often misled by the media into believing that every baby, no matter how sick or small, can become a miracle baby. Parents under the sway of feature stories of births of quadruplets, quintuplets, and higher multiples never learn—because the media fail to tell them—how dangerous these pregnancies and births are for babies and mothers and how sick and disabled the babies are as they grow.

Sometimes media hyperbole focuses on a single micropreemie—"The Size of a Coke Can!"—or on a baby whose radical surgery—"Infant Heart, the Size of a Walnut, Rebuilt and Running"—stands as testimony to a surgeon's technical prowess but not to what constitutes an appropriate reaction to nature's inevitable anatomical mistakes.

Sometimes outsiders—hospital officials, government officials, various kinds of activists with agendas of their own (people who one father characterized as "cling-ons")—force aggressive interventions on babies.

When this occurs, something perverse happens to the benefit-to-risk ratio, which is so crucial to rational decision making in the NICU. This ratio should consider whether the benefits outweigh the risks and burdens for the baby and the family. But in circumstances when interventions are imposed by others, the benefits of intervening—personal, emotional, professional, political, financial—all seem to go to the outsiders. The risks and burdens—personal, medical, emotional, social, and financial—all end up going to the babies and their families.

Some of the financial burdens do, eventually, spill over to the wider community as babies grow and remain needy. Often, schools and the medical and social services in the local community are not fully prepared to meet the children's unique needs, and this can create additional problems for both the family and the community.

Chapter 7

Quality of Life Matters

TRUTH-TELLING

Why the communities are so ill-prepared to proactively assist with the needs of sick children may be directly related to how deeply hidden the lives and struggles of these children and their families are. Lavish attention is showered on vulnerable babies when they are born, but as the children grow, they and their parents founder on their own, dealing with crises and seeking medical and educational services and help.

What do outsiders actually hear and know about sick and disabled children? What information is included, and what is excluded, from the storytellers' narratives?

Neonatologists share their clinical findings—tell their stories—with one another in the medical literature. They describe discoveries and accomplishments—almost always incremental rather than monumental—and this allows other neonatal intensivists, doctors, and nurses to ponder the lessons learned and the relevance of the information to their own clinical practices. Journalists also read the medical literature. All of these readers pass along take-home messages to others.

As stories are retold and broadcast, they can change. The process sometimes resembles the children's game "telephone," in which a story metamorphoses as it moves from child to child. Children expect to smile and laugh at the end of their game, knowing that the story will be hopelessly muddled through the retelling.

Sometimes, when the stories of the lives of sick children are retold, they too make audiences smile, but that happens because, in the retelling, painful facts get dropped, emphases shift, and the story might even take on the proverbial happy ending. The casualty here is truth.

In early 2006, for example, a group of neonatologists and their research collaborators published the latest in a continuing series of "outcome" studies that they have been conducting and publishing on the developmental milestones of a group of extremely low birth weight (ELBW) preemies who were born in Ontario, Canada, between 1977 and 1982. At the quarter-century mark, the researchers were asking how well the 149 ex-preemies—90 percent of the original group—and the normal-birth-weight children in the control group were making the transition from adolescence to young adulthood.

The researchers interviewed the ex-preemies and the controls. But if the ex-preemie was "severely impaired and unable to respond," then they interviewed the parents. They examined how far each individual had gone in school, whether they were working or had continued on to college, whether they were living independently, and whether they were married and having children.

The *Journal of the American Medical Association* published the nine-page article, which included five tables and lengthy explanations of the research methods, the data, and the authors' interpretations of the findings.

The journal also published in that issue a careful critique of the study by U.S. researchers, who compared the Canadian data with their own continuing study of ex-preemies born in Cleveland, Ohio.

The Cleveland results have, over the years, been less positive than the Canadian findings. The U.S. researchers attributed the differences to socioeconomic, societal, and family differences in the two cohorts of ex-preemies. The Canadian children were mostly white, grew up in two-parent "advantaged" homes, and had the benefits of a supportive National Health system. More than half of the children in the Cleveland group were black, most were poor and urban, and most of their mothers were single.

"The fact that the Canadian ELBW young adults functioned as well as they did seems mainly due to contextual factors," wrote the U.S. commentators. "However, even the most optimal societal and environmental benefits cannot 'fix' the enormous biological risk associated with extremely low birth weight. . . . The Canadians who graduated from high school, even those without neurosensory impairments, were significantly less likely to complete the requirements for university entrance and fewer were enrolled in or had completed their university education at age twenty-three years. Furthermore, more ELBW young adults than controls were neither occupied in study nor work, mainly due to chronic illness or permanent disability. Male ELBW young adults had poorer educational outcomes . . . and they worked in un-skilled and semi-skilled jobs rather than management . . ."

Within two weeks of the publication of the data and the commentary, the story made its way into the popular press. By then, though, most of the bad news was missing or buried. The headline published by the *New York Times*, for example, was "Achievement of Preemies is Found to be Near Normal." The *Washington Post* titled its coverage "In Canada, Preemies Seem to Catch Up Later in Life."

Deeper in the *Times* story was a line about the proxy answers given by parents of those ex-preemies too disabled to speak and about the special vul-nerability of ELBW males; buried in the *Post* coverage was a sentence ex-plaining that the "mental and/or physical disabilities related to their prema-ture births" explained why 39 percent of ELBW preemies were neither in school nor employed.

Neither article mentioned that the employment of some of the ex-preemies was at sheltered workshops, that some were living in group homes or assisted-living facilities, and that eight individuals who had refused to participate in the study had serious neurosensory impairments—autism, cerebral palsy, and cognitive dysfunctions.

These and other downbeat facts had been included in the original article. Still, neither the authors nor the editors of the journal selected them for the pickup, single-sentence, "bottom-line" conclusion of the article's abstract: "Our study results indicate that a significant majority of former ELBW infants have overcome their earlier difficulties to become functional young adults."

EDWARD

Misrepresentations of the quality of the lives of rescued preemies—in both the popular press and also in many articles in the primary medical literature—

have exasperated parents of preemies for some time. For example, Helen Harrison, author of *The Premature Baby Book* and chief architect of "The Principles," told me that, on the basis of the criteria and research methods used in the Canadian studies, her son Edward's enrollment in the school for retarded children could be listed as "post graduate" education and that Edward would be considered to have made "a successful transition to adulthood."

Edward is slightly older than the ex-preemies in the Canadian study group: he recently celebrated his thirtieth birthday. He is a man, physically— five feet six inches tall and weighing 160 pounds.

Edward wakes up each morning with a scrubby beard that needs to be shaved. But shaving Edward's beard is something that his parents must do for him. He also cannot brush his own teeth or take a shower or use the bathroom by himself. He attends a school for retarded children, where he is the oldest student and the only one with physical as well as cognitive disabilities. He has little depth perception, but he can read large print; his reading preferences lie with *Berenstain Bear* books.

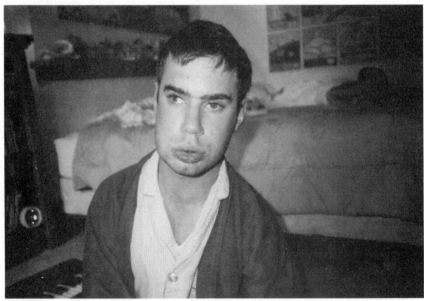

Helen Harrison

Edward at twenty-nine. He is retarded and autistic and has cerebral palsy and severe vision impairment.

Edward walks with a marked limp, but he can't go anywhere by himself. He spends hours each day listening to the radio and to cassettes; he is not dextrous enough to manage CDs. He can compose music on his keyboard, and he plays tunes flawlessly, albeit with one finger.

Edward's speech is unclear, and he can't reliably answer yes-and-no questions. Yet he can communicate, at times inventively. When Edward was in the hospital to have a cavity filled, for example—a procedure that required general anesthesia and which Helen referred to as "Edward's $20,000 cavity"—he sang the Stones' song "Let it Bleed" and the Coasters' song "Poison Ivy" to let his parents know that his mouth had been bleeding and that he'd had an intravenous (IV) line.

OUTCOME MYTHOLOGIES

Some years ago, Helen critiqued one of the earlier reports about the progress of the ELBW ex-preemies in an article that she titled "Making Lemonade: A Parent's View of 'Quality of Life' Studies."[1]

One of the report's most egregious claims, Helen noted, but not the only one, was that the quality of life was rated as perfect by 61 percent of the ex-preemies, (compared with 49 percent for the controls). Yet in the group of ex-preemies were teens who were blind, teens who could not walk, and teens with various other serious impairments. She found the researchers' survey methods flawed and their conclusions at odds with easily observed objective measures of the children's actual quality of life.

Helen was frustrated knowing that neonatologists who read this paper would use the rosy outcome data "to provide optimistic counsel to new and prospective parents of extremely premature infants."

Parents knew differently, she told me. Even the principal investigator of the Canadian study admitted that 94 percent of her colleagues in neonatology would not want aggressive care for their own newborn, if the child would be likely to survive with impairments. Helen suspected that the study's chief value was to provide "reassurance to professionals who might otherwise be dispirited by reports of worsening outcomes among extremely low birth weight survivors."

---

[1] Helen Harrison, "Making Lemonade: A Parent's View of 'Quality of Life' Studies," *Journal of Clinical Ethics*, 2001, 12(3): 239–250.

Other parents of ex-preemies had reacted with similar disbelief and anger to that earlier study. Twelve of them sent a group letter to the editor of the *Journal of the American Medical Association*, critiquing the 1996 quality-of-life assessments this way:

"As parents and family members of severely disabled children, we find the scenarios . . . presented for quality of life evaluations to be out of touch with the harsh realities of our children's lives. Where is the description of the months or years of grueling hospitalizations with the associated gastrostomy tubes, jejunostomy tubes, and fundoplications; the tracheostomies, shunts, and orthopedic, eye, and brain surgeries; hyperalimentation, oxygen tanks, and ventilators? Similarly, there was no mention of bankruptcies, divorces, mental and physical breakdowns, deaths in late childhood, neglected siblings, and suicides caused by the extreme burdens of caring for severely medically and developmentally compromised children."[2]

These parents, enduring so much hardship in their lives with their sick and disabled children, were dismayed that the researchers would so misrepresent the quality of their lives and so readily dismiss their suffering and the suffering of their children. Why weren't the intensivists facing and accepting the grim realities that the parents had been forced to face and accept every hour since their babies were born and rescued? And why weren't the intensivists willing to be truthful when they talked to future parents?

That letter's signatories felt—as had the producers of the BBC documentary *When Miracle Baby Grows Up*—that, if new parents were given accurate and honest information about outcomes and about what life could be like for families and babies born at risk, not all parents would blithely choose to plunge forward in pursuit of nonstop heroics.

Helen interpreted the self-reported positive ratings of the ex-preemies in the study group to be expedient coping mechanisms common to many children and their parents who live with these difficult realities.

"Upon becoming parents of a disabled or 'high-risk' child, one of the first things we learn to do is lie—to our friends and family, to the doctors, to our child, and to ourselves. We quickly learn that others do not want an honest answer when they ask, 'How are you (or your child) doing?' and we oblige

---

[2] Gloria Culver et al, letter to the editor, "Informed Decisions for Extremely Low-Birth-Weight Infants," *Journal of the American Medical Association*, 2000, 283(24): 3201.

by giving the positive and politically correct answer . . . We don't lie just to reassure others. An arguably more important motive is the need to comfort ourselves and give positive meaning to the immense physical and emotional difficulties of our lives. . . . We are 'special parents' to 'special children.' We lie to deny, or at least postpone unpleasant realities. We believe that our children's problems can be overcome with therapies, interventions, and, of course, the 'right' parental attitude. If we play our role with bravery, all might end happily. We try to raise the self-esteem of those of our children who are able to understand the concept, by reminding them of their heroic fight for life and by encouraging them to accept and embrace their 'challenges' with pride. . . . Eventually most children with disabilities, like their parents, learn to put on a brave public face . . . The comforting lies (or failure to tell the uncomfortable truth) are not simply emotional coping mechanisms for many of us. They are practical necessities if we want our children to get proper medical and educational services. . . . We who are parents of children with disabilities . . . use multiple versions of the truth on a daily basis. There is the truth we acknowledge in private, and there is 'making lemonade'—the brave face we instinctively offer to the public."

How easy, Helen said to me, would it be for a child or a parent to grumble about an outcome to the very physicians who saved that child's life?

OUTCOMES

Outcome studies are absolutely essential. They are guides for the future. They establish which interventions are effective and which ones don't work or, worse, cause harm.

The big picture of what was happening to the children in the EPICure study, for example—so many children growing up with so many disabilities—helped British and Dutch and other neonatologists rethink their nonstop push toward the rescue of younger and younger preemies, and they changed both their NICU procedures and their policies.

Outcome data can be helpful not just for future babies but also for those who are being studied, if they motivate and guide policy makers and communities toward providing the medical, educational, social, and other services that the study participants need.

If outcome data are accurately reported by the media, they can raise public awareness of the existence of children who were born at risk and of the challenges facing their families and perhaps lead to improvements in the quality of their lives. The New Zealand families, for example, were requesting inclusion in, rather than marginalization from, activities that other families were enjoying.

Outcome data are, though, only valuable if researchers ask the right questions, if they listen closely to the answers, if they do not hide or overlook discouraging results, and if they and those who hear and read their stories relay the findings truthfully to others.

Researchers and the media must be willing to describe how all of the children are doing as they grow, not just the ones who are doing well. When they ignore bad news or pass on a misleading or falsely reassuring take-home message, then outcome data help no one (except, perhaps, the storytellers). False reporting exacerbates the problems, not just for existing children and their families, but also for future families, by suggesting that the problems of high-risk births and sick and disabled children are just temporary.

A continuing enigma associated with outcome data is how relevant data from NICU practices of one, two, or three decades ago are to NICU practices today. Interventions, treatments, technologies, drugs, and procedures change all the time.

Siva told me that most neonatologists of the 1970s and 1980s were "technicians," but that by the 1990s most were focusing more on being "healers." They kept looking for less invasive approaches for caring for babies. For example, they began then to use C-PAP for babies who were having trouble breathing because this device is less damaging than ventilators, which so often jeopardize the integrity and functioning of the babies' fragile lungs and blood vessels.

Neonatologists continually investigate, tabulate, and parse good outcomes, bad outcomes, and their significance. They mull over the implications of their data and consider how to modify their daily medical practices. None of this is easy or straightforward. They face an enormous challenge—how to innovate and still be safe.

But as hard as these tasks are for neonatologists, their relations with outcomes are infinitely easier than are families'. Families actually live outcomes. They are called "lives."

Chapter 8

Coping with Complexity

GRAHAM

"Margaret and I continue to occasionally feel exasperated that we are still providing significant medical care for Graham," Lawrence said to me recently.

"Our lounge can still sometimes resemble an Outpatients Department with all of the equipment he requires. There really is no end to this in sight, and we're getting close to his eleventh birthday! Still, Graham continues to inspire and frustrate me in equal measure."

Graham was born at 27 weeks gestation weighing one pound and three ounces, his eyes were still fused shut, and his ears did not yet have cartilage. He was given a 5 percent chance to survive, and his parents were told that, if he did survive, the likelihood of his having disabilities was between 5 and 85 percent. Graham spent the first six months of his life in the NICU.

I have not met Graham, but I spoke at length to both of his parents on the telephone. And I have seen pictures of this spirited boy—shiny blond hair, bright eyes, big smile, often mugging for the camera. The family lives in England, and both parents are deeply involved with and committed to their engaging, unique, and complex son. (I have substituted names for these parents and their son at their request.)

"Graham is very outgoing and confident one-on-one," Margaret said. "Sometimes when people meet him they think he is just fine."

"He's all personality," Lawrence said, "full of energy and a zest for life. He's a really happy kid."

Graham can read words, but often he can't comprehend what he is reading. He might grasp some of the peripheral information, but he isn't really able to identify a central theme. His handwriting is poor, and his grasp of math is "a nightmare." He speaks with a heavy stammer, his language is quite delayed, and he often has difficulty retrieving words. Sometimes he can get halfway through a sentence, and then he can't find the rest of the words he needs. He has to work "bloody hard," his father said, to get his school work done.

Graham walks into things because he cannot glance.

"On a good day, you look at him," Lawrence said, "and you think he can make it. On other days, he can hardly cross the road. He has every right to be pretty miserable with his life, but he isn't. He now is at an age where he realizes he is a bit different. But he's just fantastic. Our friends say he has been put on the planet to teach us, rather than to learn. It's easy to get new-agey about him."

"Having a child who is so complicated developmentally made me someone I wouldn't normally be," Margaret said, "especially because care for chronic problems is not at the same high standard as acute care is in the National Health Service. Our acute care is fabulous. But mums and dads are forced afterward to be advocates. I'm a lot more driven than I once was. I go kicking doors down. I have no doubt that I have a reputation because I say, 'You saved this child, but that's not good enough. Now he needs an education.'

"It is incomprehensible to have a child in the NICU. It's all so acute, life or death, hour by hour. The 'miracle baby' that the media talks about is crap. They leave you with an expectation, a hope. And that's not fair.

"I was so very driven to understand how to support Graham when he was in the NICU. We wanted him to know us. We would make tapes or sleep with hankies and put them in his incubator. I was absolutely desperate to get messages to him."

Margaret and Lawrence both talked about a wonderful NICU nurse who worked closely with them, guided them as they learned how to care for their

son, and served as their "interpreter," explaining what the doctors were doing and what they were trying to achieve.

"I can't see why people think preemies will come through unscathed,"
Margaret said. "How can people who have a preemie believe that the baby will
be fine? There's a reason pregnancy is forty weeks. Yet some people genuinely
think their child will catch up. Preemies don't catch up. 'Moving on' is a better term. They move on, but they never fully leave their prematurity behind."

"I was working twelve or fourteen hours a day when Graham was born,"
Lawrence said, "wanting the whole thing—the manager job, the company
car, etc. I didn't know much biology then, although one of my A-levels was
in biology. But with a child in the NICU, you get hungry for information. I
think I'm reasonably medicalized now. Graham made me think that it's
unimportant to have a brand new car in the driveway. I'm happy just to be
at home with my family. Show me a person who isn't completely changed by
being a father and I'll show you an idiot."

When Graham got home from the NICU with oxygen tanks and a gas-
tronomy tube (G tube) that stayed in for six years, Margaret stopped working to care full time for their son. (She had been trained in the law.)

"When Graham was a baby, I'd absent myself in the evenings," Margaret
said. "So at night, Lawrence was the main caregiver. And what we have today
is a child who, at age ten, sees that his parents can respond to him equally."

Lawrence said, "My position in the early days was that I'd do whatever
we had to in order to help him survive. We made a conscious effort at the beginning to share in Graham's care. I always wanted to be the kind of father
who did more than just a share of cooking . . . changing nappies, teaching
values. And I'd say my relationship with Graham now is quite sparky; we
tend to be really, really good mates or we spat at each other."

"We came very close to splitting up at one point," Margaret said. "The
situation was making us tired, and fatigue makes you act sarcastically and in
obnoxious ways. We stopped making sound judgments. Exhaustion makes
you do terrible things."

"Work was a welcome relief for me," Lawrence said. "The adrenaline you
get from work is helpful, and it's a distraction. I didn't have time during the day
to think about anything outside work. Going to work probably kept me sane."

Some people knew how to give support to Margaret and Lawrence, but
not everyone.

"You learn which people you can discuss things with," Lawrence said, "and you whittle down your list. Lots of people tell you stories, like 'Oh, my friend had a tiny baby and she did so well.' But for each of these, there are plenty of stories of a child who is deaf, blind, living in an institution with no quality of life. I would just nod and walk off and think 'you're an idiot.'

"At work I still find it difficult when people come in and complain about their sick child who has kept them up all night with an ear infection. Our reality is so different from theirs. Everything is relative.

"We have an expression over here when people are having children—you ask, 'Are you having a boy or girl?' And people will say, 'I don't care as long as it's healthy.' And I say back to them: 'And what if the baby is not healthy? If your child isn't well it does not alter your love for him.'

"There was a newborn in the office recently, a really chubby baby. And everyone was oohing and aahing and saying, 'We love chubby babies.' And I said, 'Trust me, there's nothing wrong with the skinny babies.' In the first year, Graham looked like a bird who had fallen out of the nest. For us, that's what was 'normal'—the little ones—those are the ones we cooed over."

(A NICU nurse told me something similar. She said that in her unit "we get so used to tiny babies that full-term newborns look like Sumo babies—in fact, we actually call them Sumo babies! And we prefer the teeny tinies.")

"People are a little bit naïve, ignorant," Lawrence said. "They use insulting language. For example, they might say something about their 'normal' child. How bloody dare they? Their thoughtlessness can hurt.

"My focus has always been on Graham. In the beginning, we had no idea what to expect. We were told there was only a small chance Graham would survive, and within that, they expected he would be blind, deaf, etc. When you look at him against that backdrop, it's remarkable what he's achieved.

"Still, I'm more pessimistic now about his future than Margaret is; I wonder, for example, if he is ever going to hold down a job. He simply doesn't 'get' things. For example, someone asked him if he has a brother or a sister, and he said yes, he had a brother and a sister. When we asked him about it, he said, 'What about Catherine and Gerrold?' They are his cousins. It's odd for a ten-year-old not to know whether he has siblings.

"I have never been one for introspection. I'm a typical Englishman: You've got to get on with it. If I sit and cry in the corner, I'm not helping anyone. There might be a time in my life when I will do that, but it hasn't come so far."

Lawrence said that, around the time that Graham was two months old, he and Margaret were driving home from the hospital talking about what they hoped for. Both had graduated from university, and they had always assumed that any child of theirs would do that too. But they realized that this child probably would not follow their trajectories. They agreed that, as long as their son grew up happy, it didn't matter what he did. They would be content if he would just grow up.

"When our friend said that Graham was not here to learn but to teach people something, a shiver went down my spine," Lawrence said. "I'm not a religious or spiritual person. But there is something in him that is remarkable. We can't believe this is his first time on the planet. Something in his eyes makes us think he's been here before.

"There's a kind of knowledge that he has. He's wise, but also massively innocent, tremendously stupid. He's just not grounded. It's like he's floating around, occasionally here, then floating around, then he comes back down into his body.

"You know when you are sitting in a classroom and all of a sudden you've lost the thread of the lecture, and you think that you don't have a clue what's going on and you think everyone else does? I think Graham may feel that a lot. He puts his hand up all the time in school, but he may not have a clue what the answer to the question is. I don't know if he knows himself. I can't say that I know him. But he's really intriguing.

"What I am trying to do is help him find his own way, to become the best he can become. He's a remarkable boy. He knows he's loved. We have been very conscious to tell him that every day."

ELLY

"Elly is inherently medical," Wendy Greathouse told me. "We aren't interested in 'fixing' Elly as she isn't broken. We are interested in keeping the demons of sickness at bay.

"Knowing that Elly is predisposed to certain illnesses simply because she has a chromosome deletion is heartrending. Goodness, there's a lot to deal with just with the 'typical' genetic background that we have passed on to our two other kids."

Elly was not, like Graham, a preemie. She was born at full term on February 1, 2002. She was one day old when the family pediatrician discovered that she had a cleft palate. A month later, Elly was rehospitalized with a dangerous viral infection—respiratory syncytial virus—and it was then that the doctors began noticing developmental delays and atypical anatomic features.

Elly spent eight days on a ventilator. Then the family pediatrician sent Elly for what Wendy described as a slew of services—a genetics work up, a meeting with a speech therapist, a consult with a physical therapist, a session with an occupational therapist, and various other evaluations. The geneticist discovered that Elly had a rare anomaly, a spontaneous deletion in the Q37 region of chromosome #2. Just thirty-four other children around the world were known at the time to have that specific deletion.

"Elly's first genetics appointment was difficult to get through," Wendy said the first time we talked. "She is a beautiful little girl, with no obvious physical defects." So it was wrenching to listen as the doctors rattled off a menacing and largely incomprehensible list of physical and physiological anomalies—aberrant right subclavian artery off a left aortic arch, macrocephaly, micrognathia, mild Pierre Robin sequence, hypertelorism, mild midface hypoplasia, cerebral hypotonia, mild microtia, anteverted nares, antimongoloid palpebral fissures, simian crease, frontal bossing, long tapered fingers and toes, cleft of the soft palate.

"In a strange twist of fate," Wendy told me, "I have always loved genetics, ever since my fifth grade science fair project on Mendel's peas." Thus, with Elly's diagnosis, Wendy decided that "it was incumbent on me to figure out what the repercussions of these missing pieces are, and I plunged headfirst into the field of genetics. I found a large number of proteins and enzymes which, theoretically, have been disrupted because of Elly's chromosome deletion.

"Elly has always been a placid child. She can stay in one place, without human interaction, for hours on end. She is generally unruffled. Her life sweeps by, and as long as no one pokes at her or offers too much in-your-face stimulation, she doesn't give a fig. Even when we know that something is painful or problematic, Elly evidences no discomfort."

When Elly was one year old, she began having seizures. She would tire easily, and she didn't babble the way a typical one-year-old does. Still, she

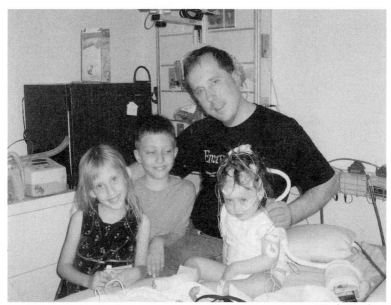

Wendy Greathouse

Elly at the clinic having an EEG of her brain; her dad and siblings at her side.

would giggle appropriately, reach for objects, and her emotions spanned a standard range—anger to glee.

By the time Elly was three, she had become "hypersocial," chatting with "anyone anywhere for any reason." She liked men the best; Wendy thought perhaps she was responding to the lower pitches of their voices.

Wendy described Elly then as "a traffic stopper: great big blue eyes, a mop of chestnut hair that curls slightly at the ends, and porcelain skin when her body is working correctly." Her skin had "the kind of pink and white complexion that expensive dolls have, but rarely children."

By the time Elly was four, she was walking and "talking around her trache," a tracheostomy tube that had been inserted in her neck to help her breathe when she was sixteen months old. She was taking dance classes, was beginning to enjoy playing "pretend," and was an active participant in fights with her older sister and brother.

"On good days," Wendy said, "Elly can recognize colors and numbers; on good days, she can use pronouns, verbs, and proper tenses." And usually Elly's personality is "very sunny. She has a wicked sense of humor, and she's

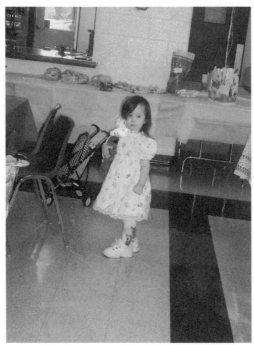

Wendy Greathouse
Elly with her tracheostomy tube and leg braces

a good mimic. She can copy people, and she understands how to make people laugh. She has an excellent memory."

But at four, Elly is still being fed through a G tube at night, and she still cannot drink liquids. And for unknown reasons and uncharacteristically for a child with a 2Q37 deletion, Elly has begun regressing in certain ways. She has developed a "wibbly-wobbly" gait, which means that she "could just as easily stagger right into a wall as go through the doorway." She also has been less able than in the past to plan her movements: "Sometimes she can climb onto a couch with no problems," Wendy said, "but at other times the couch might as well be Mount Rushmore."

Elly, like Debby Barrett's son Michael, cannot recognize danger. "You have to tell her," Wendy said, "that it isn't safe to push the screen out the door, or climb out the window, or put her hand in the dog's mouth, or sit on the stove, or turn the gas on."

Around Thanksgiving in 2005, the family went to the National Human Genome Research Institute at the National Institutes of Health (NIH) to participate in a genetics study. They drove from Ohio to Maryland and stayed at the Children's Inn, which is affiliated with the NIH.

Wendy and Elly spent an entire day going from clinic to clinic, lab to lab, getting various tests and diagnoses. The researchers took blood samples from Wendy and her husband Ken, and they made three-dimensional pictures of Elly's sister and brother to help them sort out which of Elly's physical features are and are not associated with the missing genes.

"The visit to NIH was lovely," Wendy told me. "We were not there for a medical reason, so it wasn't stressful. It didn't really matter what the results were."

The geneticists are interested in identifying exactly which genes Elly is missing. They expect, eventually, to correlate Elly's specific clinical problems with the missing activities of the missing genes. They hope to gain a basic understanding of how the genes in the Q37 region function and what goes awry when individual genes are absent.

Elly will not, as Wendy said, get any direct genetic benefits from the study. But indirectly she will benefit from the thorough medical workup she had there. Her parents are learning more about their daughter's distinctive physiology, anatomy, and metabolism. They also now know more things to look out for and which specialists need to be following Elly regularly in order to forestall other problems that might arise as a result of the 2Q37 deletions.

The researchers are hoping to learn also which of Elly's problems are unique to her and which ones may be common to other children with 2Q37 deletions. Such information could help other clinicians treat and advise other children with this anomaly.

"As tiring as Elly's problems are," Wendy said, "we're lucky to have her. She's not what we would have chosen, but she has been fun. She has refocused us on the family and redefined us.

"She has taught the big kids some things about people. They have learned some social graces—they know now how to talk to people who are staring at Elly.

"Her presence has also helped them to become self-reliant. If Elly is sick, her health comes first, and we end up doing what the other kids need versus what they want. But we don't neglect their activities; she doesn't stop their lives.

"We hope that someday Elly will be able to read. But I don't know. She's not autistic yet, but we now know that seventy-five percent of the kids with this deletion are.

"Some days we are getting through it; other days we are having fun. We go a day at a time."

And what about the nights? "I don't really sleep at night," Wendy said. "I listen for alarms."

CHLOE

"Chloe is the happiest baby you ever saw," Becky Means told me when Chloe was two years old. "That is, ninety-nine percent of the time. But when she's mad, look out! You can't force her to do anything she doesn't want to do."

Chloe was a "fighting twenty pounds" when I first talked to Becky, and although Chloe instinctively grasped what was involved in the infamous terrible twos concept, she was functioning at a ten-month level, and she looked more like a one-year-old. She was attending a school for medically fragile and developmentally disabled children, where she received physical, occupational, and speech therapy. She couldn't chew or swallow, so she, like Elly, was fed through a G tube.

Becky and her husband Corey learned that something was amiss with their first child just four hours before she was born on August 25, 2000. The fetal monitor detected a decreasing heart rate. Then, a sonogram showed that the fetus was small for a full-term baby (three pounds and eight ounces) and that she was surrounded by fluid. The sonogram also suggested that the fetus had a cleft lip and palate.

"Those are red flags for chromosome anomalies," Becky said, but when Chloe was born the doctor's first reaction was, "Oh, no. She's fine."

The NICU staff went back and forth during the first few weeks of Chloe's life trying to decide if her problems were genetic. Eventually they found that Chloe had a chromosome anomaly.

Chloe's anomaly was what Becky termed "a fluke." Chloe had not inherited the altered chromosome from either parent; during her development, some genes in the Q arm of chromosome #3 had erroneously gotten dupli-

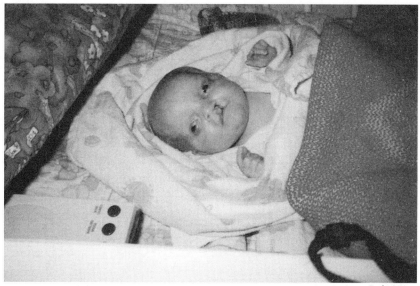

Becky Means

Chloe at birth

cated. (Or, as the father of another child I spoke with put it—the Gods of the Odds duplicated some genes.)

Just forty other children were known at the time, throughout the world, to have that same anomaly. Seventy-five percent of them inherited the duplication from a parent. Their syndrome is called pseudo Cornelia de Lange. But Chloe's version of the de Lange syndrome has been atypical all along.

"At first I asked 'why me?'" Becky said. "It was pretty devastating. I didn't do drugs, drink. I didn't even eat chocolate because of the caffeine. I said— this doesn't happen to people like me." But of course it does.

"Corey and I totally believe we had Chloe for a reason," Becky said, "but we'll probably never know what that reason is."

Becky and Corey had gotten strong support from the NICU staff in their town—Springfield, Missouri. The nurses and doctors had worked hard to get Chloe ready to go home so that Becky and Corey could enjoy as much time as possible with their baby. All of the other babies with pseudo de Lange syndrome had died by age one, and the doctors predicted that Chloe would do the same.

"You pull yourself up, dust yourself off," Becky said. "You learn to be thankful for what you have. You can live in misery or live each day. I was not gonna wallow in it. Two of my friends had worse problems. One had a still-born baby, and then she had another baby with a congenital lung problem. Another friend had one baby who had anencephaly, and then she had twins, both of whom died.

"That first year, I was obsessed with the Internet," Becky said. "We were in uncharted territory. I would stay up until two or three in the morning looking for information."

Becky discovered the Unique website, where parents of children with unique genetic anomalies could find one another. (Wendy, too, was very involved with Unique, as well as the Chromosome Deletion Outreach group).

"The biggest benefit of Unique was just knowing that there are others out there dealing with this weird stuff," Becky said. "The newsletter made me feel that maybe Chloe is not so bad off, and also that she might be able to achieve certain things."

At the time of our first conversation, Becky was in the midst of a number of time-consuming negotiations. Chloe needed a $4,000 wheelchair. "We have a decent income, but it's not enough," she said. "If we spend that much for a wheelchair for Chloe, our other child will suffer." Chloe's little sister, Carly Jane, was just three months old at the time.

Becky was also trying to get reimbursed for Chloe's seven cleft lip and palate surgeries. This battle began when an agent at the insurance company had labeled those surgeries "cosmetic."

"Chloe needs special education, special equipment, and so on, and I have to do all this footwork," Becky said. "Healthy kids: they just go to school. The mother doesn't have to find everything on her own.

"God must be someone with a sense of humor to pick me—someone with no patience—to have a child who requires so much patience. I have a lot of patience with Chloe, but with no one else."

Becky, like Wendy, had enrolled Chloe in a genetics study, this one at the Children's Hospital of Pennsylvania. "I would do anything to take away Chloe's genetic problem," Becky said, "but Chloe is always going to be Chloe. The CHOP study won't help her, but it might help other children in the future.

"Chloe's development has been a big fat question. We were told originally that she would probably die by her first birthday. The other forty children with pseudo de Lange syndrome had. But now we are being told that she'll have a normal life span."

When Chloe was three years old and I spoke again to Becky, Chloe still weighed twenty pounds, and she was thirty inches tall. She had begun to say a few words—hi, bye, mama—and she was doing some signing. Meantime, Carly Jane was also saying mama and dada and beginning to serve as a role model for her big sister.

Becky was training a service dog, Rudy, a German shepherd, a descendent of Rin Tin Tin. He would eventually be able to pull Chloe's wheelchair and perhaps help her gain some independence. Becky loved and admired dogs. She talked about the golden retriever she and Corey had when Chloe was born. That dog had mostly ignored the new baby. But whenever Chloe was in trouble or started to get sick, she would go to Chloe's side and stay there, as though alerting them that Chloe needed attention.

Chloe got really sick during her third winter. She had unending infections and fevers. She gained only three ounces the whole year. She began having seizures, she coded—stopped breathing and had to be resuscitated—several times. Images of her brain indicated that certain structures were smaller than they should be. This, too, was typical for a child with her chromosome anomaly.

A turning point came that year when a dietician suggested a new liquid diet for her. Within one month, Chloe gained eight pounds.

Around that time, the governor of Missouri proposed abolishing the state's First Steps Program, which provides services for children, like Chloe, who have severe mental and physical handicaps. Becky drove to a hearing in Jefferson City and was interviewed by a reporter from the *Kansas City Star*. She was quoted as saying that she was "sick" that the governor wanted to eliminate the program: "Because of the intense therapy, we are finally hearing Chloe's first words . . . It meant that she was able to stay home and be raised by her family rather than being placed in an institution . . . We really feel being pro-life means a lot more than saving babies from abortions. You also help those who can't mentally and physically take care of themselves. We feel like these kids are getting swept under the rug."

"I felt really discriminated against personally just once," Becky told me. "That was when Chloe was an infant and some friends paid a babysitting

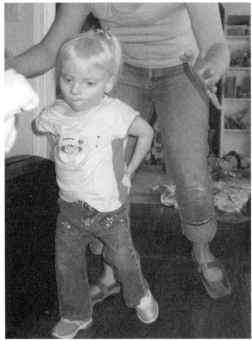

Becky Means
Chloe takes her first step at age five and one-half

service so that I could have some time out. But the service wouldn't do it. People are afraid of the G tube, but they were more scared of Chloe when they heard she is retarded."

Now Chloe is five and one-half. She is still small: she weighs twenty-eight pounds, and she is thirty-three inches tall. She walks with a walker that supports her from the back. Rudy is no longer with them. Becky said he "got bored with Chloe," because there wasn't much he could do for her. So they gave him to a teenager in Ohio who has cerebral palsy and could benefit from his support and companionship.

Chloe's overall development is now between that of a twelve-month-old and an eighteen-month-old. Her receptive learning is somewhat higher than that, and she is able to handle more stimulation now than she has in the past. But she still needs complete structure in her life.

"If she's overstimulated," Becky said, "she falls apart. When that happens, we say she's humpty-dumptying, and there is absolutely nothing we can do."

Becky and Corey took Chloe, Carly Jane, and the baby Landree to the zoo recently, and they were pleased that Chloe did well. On outings like this and on longer trips, Becky carries what she calls The Bag of Life—extra formula, resuscitation equipment, a stethoscope, medicines, and a community advance directive, a do-not-resuscitate order.

"I've known about advance directives for a long time," Becky said. "I was a communications major in college. We studied various stories that were reported in the media, like the story of Nancy Cruzan. In fact, when Chloe was born and on a ventilator and having the G tube inserted, we made sure that they could take her off the ventilator should something go wrong in the surgery. We didn't want her to be stuck in a shell of a body.

"When Chloe coded in the hospital earlier this year, the staff was right there to resuscitate her. But when she coded at home, it took some time for the ambulance to arrive. Corey and I decided to write a community do-not-resuscitate order for paramedics but not one for the hospital. Should Chloe stop breathing again for a long time—before the paramedics could get here—we would not want them to resuscitate her. She's the happiest child I ever met. But she has very few skills. I wouldn't want her life to be more limited than it already is."

Chapter 9

Advance Directives

DO NOT RESUSCITATE

The idea behind a do-not-resuscitate order or any advance directive is that individuals take the time, long before a medical crisis occurs, to consider what they would want rescue personnel to do should that crisis arise. Many people think about writing advance directives as they age. Some people want to live as long as possible, no matter how limited their capacities become. Others ask not to be kept alive if they cannot enjoy the sort of life they are currently living. And, between these two extremes, every imaginable combination of preferences has been expressed.

Advance directives originate in the medical ethics concept of autonomy. People want to control what happens in their lives, even when they no longer have the capacity to express their desires. An advance directive is one way that they try to ensure that their preferences and wishes are understood and respected by others and that these preferences are not trumped by the preferences and wishes of others—doctors, nurses, paramedics, family members, and anyone else who might get involved during the medical crisis.

Media coverage of tragic clashes at the bedside—such as those that occurred during the long dying of Terri Schiavo from 1990 to 2005, Nancy Cruzan from 1983 to 1990 (her story is the one that Becky mentioned—she was in a persistent vegetative state in Missouri until the U.S. Supreme Court agreed that her parents had the right to ask that her feeding tube be removed), and others—have raised awareness, even among some young adults, that writing an advance directive for oneself is important.

As painful and heartbreaking as it is for parents to think about, writing an advance directive for an at-risk child, like Chloe, also makes good sense.

PRENATAL ADVANCE DIRECTIVES

Similarly wrenching is the concept of a prenatal advance directive, a kind of pre-negotiated treatment plan for an imperiled newborn. But it, too, is wise. So often, the end of life occurs just minutes, or hours, or days after a life begins. For most future parents, the thought of writing an advance directive before a child is even born seems unthinkable, yet doing that is perhaps one of the most thoughtful things they could do for their unborn child.

Anita Catlin, who developed the palliative care protocol with Brian Carter, has been developing a template for prenatal advance directives and pushing the concept within the nursing and medical communities. She points out that such directives would help parents understand their preferences should their baby be born prematurely or sick. In working through the process of articulating their wishes, future parents would also learn what is feasible and what is not.

"Parents in the United States are directly involved in making choices of care for their critically ill newborns," wrote Anita in "Thinking Outside the Box: Prenatal Care and the Call for a Prenatal Advance Directive" in 2005,[1] "yet most often have had no prenatal education to prepare them. Not knowing that twenty-seven weeks may be needed to ensure lung development or vessel integrity, parents plead for technological support for their twenty-two week fetuses. Fetal development necessary for a healthy viability and survival without impairment has never been explained to them. . . .

"Much of the education women receive about preterm delivery occurs at the bedside when preterm labor is occurring, or during or immediately after a preterm birth. At these critical periods, they are often asked to make seri-

---

[1] Anita Catlin, "Thinking Outside the Box: Prenatal Care and the Call for a Prenatal Advance Directive," *Journal of Perinatal and Neonatal Nursing*, 2005, 19(2): 169–176.

ous decisions. Research suggests that the immediate postpartum period may not be the best time for parents to be educated about potential problems."

"When I was a young nurse," Anita told me, "it was definitely the doctors who were overtreating. Now I think the problem is equally distributed between doctors and parents. Parents need to understand what care is medically appropriate. If they can understand what is medically correct and what is not, then they might not keep asking for 'more, more, more' when it's not good, when it can't be.

"We need to change what we offer in prenatal care. We have to talk about fetal development and viability. And we have to counteract all of the false information that parents are getting from the media."

In some ways it is astounding that most of the 500,000 women who give birth to preemies in the United States each year know so little about human development and fetal and infant viability. (The same is true of their partners and also of the 131 million women who give birth annually throughout the world.)

Schools have apparently not been teaching much "practical biology" at any level. And this has left young adults ill equipped to assess the miracle-baby, genetic-fix, and technologic-solution stories that they hear and read about.

Anita had been dismayed as she interviewed obstetricians to learn that only 5 percent of those who were providing prenatal care to women ever discussed viability with these women. And so she began lobbying nurses and doctors to take the initiative and educate future parents about fetal viability and survival. The process, Anita said, must begin at a woman's first prenatal visit to a doctor or a clinic. The discussions could use information about the current stage of development of the fetus as a springboard; from there, the conversation could naturally segue into how likely it would be for the fetus to survive if it were born that day. Discussions such as these would obviate the need for the ineffectual bedside crash courses that so many new parents receive today.

Anita also proposed that nurses and others who teach childbirth education classes address viability in their courses. These sessions typically cover wide-ranging perinatal issues—physical and psychological changes in the pregnant woman, breathing and relaxation techniques for the birth, concerns of the fathers, postnatal issues—but fetal development and survivorship and information on long-term outcomes are not currently among them. For some women, though, this approach to education will not work because their babies may be born even before their courses begin.

(Another nurse I spoke to about viability education said, "It's ethically inexcusable that we get babies out alive but not intact. I don't really know anyone today who walks a woman through what's going on or says, 'here's what your baby would be like if born now, and now, and now.' But parents need to know this.")

"Keeping certain babies alive is simply not medically appropriate," Anita said, "and the task is for everyone involved with a baby to understand that. Medicine and nursing, as professions, do not condone inflicting pain on babies, torturing them, harming them. Doctors and nurses have professional obligations, as well as personal ones, to relieve suffering rather than to cause it or enhance it."

On a recent trip, Anita visited a NICU where a baby with a very badly damaged heart was being kept alive. Seeing that baby had disturbed her. No one—no doctor, no nurse, nor the parents—was admitting the truth about the situation or thinking about the suffering of the baby. Had that baby been born elsewhere, somewhere far from a high-tech NICU, that baby would simply have been taken home to die.

"I hope you understand," Anita said to the people at the NICU, "that this life was not meant to be."

Future parents cannot know, of course, about every danger that a new baby might encounter; neonatal intensivists can't and don't know all of them either. But future parents need to realize that some complications—births of very premature babies, births of babies who are not breathing—are common, and they should also understand what can happen under the circumstances. They should find out what their options are, what the outcomes have been, and how the outcomes have affected the interests and the quality of the lives of the baby and the baby's family. Anita said that the choices that parents make *must* affirm the value of the lives of all of the members of the family—not just the new baby but also the mother, the father, and the siblings.

THINKING THE UNTHINKABLE

Helen Harrison has also been lobbying for prenatal advance directives for some time. A decade ago, she proposed that obstetricians work with future parents to develop prenatal advance directives because the discussions that writing the advance directive would engender "would encourage parents to articulate their views in advance [of a birth], determine the philosophies of their physicians, and avoid institutions and caregivers whose definitions of 'medical reasonableness' and 'best interests' do not match their own."[2]

At the 2005 Hot Topics meeting, two neonatologists from North Carolina approached Helen while she and I were talking. They knew about her work on "The Principles." They had just heard some comments she had made at the session that had just ended. What, they asked her, was her number one suggestion for improving the interpersonal climate in the NICU?

Prenatal advance directives, Helen said. Parents should write advance directives that indicated their preferences for heroic and high-tech interventions or for palliative care, should their babies be born premature or sick.

At first both doctors brushed off the idea as impossible. How could they ask anxious pregnant women and their partners to think about the possibility of having a sick child?

But literally within three minutes, something clicked in the brains of both doctors, and they each thought that the idea was terrific. As Helen pointed out to them, yes, forcing future parents to think ahead about the possible birth of a sick or premature baby would be extremely stressful for young adults looking forward to having a baby. But the idea that they would *not* think about it ahead of time was even scarier.

Advance directives clarify what parents want. They are an important step in assuring that parents' wishes will be understood by those who will be caring for their newborn baby.

But even when the parents have expressed their preferences clearly, they have to be vigilant. Sometimes advance directives are ignored, and the directives of others trump or override those of the parents.

---

[2] Helen Harrison, letter to the editor, *Journal of Perinatology*, 2001, 15(6): 522.

Chapter 10

Legislating Lives

SIDNEY

Karla Miller had pre-registered at the Woman's Hospital of Texas in Houston many months before her first baby was due. The registration process included filling out forms about her personal and medical information and her health insurance coverage.

But just as Karla began the 23rd week of her pregnancy, she seemed to be going into labor. Her doctor admitted her to the hospital on August 17, 1990, and to stop the contractions, he suggested that she could try an experimental drug, Brethine, that had not yet been approved by the Food and Drug Administration. Brethine was risky, and the doctor told Karla that it might actually kill her. Karla decided to take the drug despite the risk because she really wanted to save her pregnancy.

The obstetrician paged a consulting neonatologist who, in a somber conversation, described to Karla and her husband Mark what would happen if labor could not be stopped and the baby were born that early.

The most likely scenario was that the fetal infant would not be born alive. But if it were, the Millers would then have two options: they could hold the baby and let "nature take its course," or they could try aggressive interventions. A 22- or 23-week fetal infant was outside the limit where viability was possible, or just at the margin; and no one there had actually ever been present for the birth of so young a micropreemie.

The doctor then explained that, should the baby end up surviving, the prognosis for the future was grim: serious neurological damage, blindness, deafness, mental retardation, lung disease, cerebral palsy, and so on.

Karla got sicker as the day went on. She had a uterine infection—chorioamnionitis—that was making her dangerously and critically ill. Around midday, her obstetrician concluded that the baby had to be born that day. He switched Karla to Pitocin, a drug that is used to induce labor and birth and which would facilitate the "evacuation" of the fetus.

Karla and Mark were in agreement that they did not want heroics for their fetal infant, just comfort care. Both their obstetrician and the consulting neonatologist agreed that this decision was sound, the right one. The obstetrician said, "This is a tragic miscarriage," and the neonatologist wrote on the chart, "Parents request no extra-heroic measures be taken at this point."

When Mark told me the story he said, "We made an informed decision. We were given all of the information about causal effects. They went A-B-C-D on all the things that could go wrong for the baby: apnea, bradycardia, cerebral palsy, etc. They called our options 'aggressive care' and 'compassionate care.' In aggressive care, they would do everything to keep the baby alive. In compassionate care, they would clean the baby up, give her to Karla, and let nature take its course. With virtual certainty that the baby would have a compromised life of pain and suffering, our decision was easier: we made the 'compassionate care' choice."

But someone, who was not the baby's parents and not one of the two doctors who were involved with the parents, was unhappy with the Millers' decision. Mark was called into a conference room. A hospital administrator told him that the hospital had a corporate policy that, if a baby were born weighing more than 500 grams (1 pound and 1.6 ounces), they would resuscitate it. They wanted Mark to sign a consent form saying that he approved of that approach. Mark said he'd like to see the hospital's policy.

"They asked me if I was a lawyer, and I said 'no, do I need a lawyer?' The administrator said 'no,' and she said she would bring me the written policies.

"Karla's obstetrician told me to go and make funeral arrangements," Mark continued. "It took me about two hours. Her doctor had decided, because of Karla's blood pressure, heart rate, and spiking fever, to 'evacuate' the fetus. When I came back, the ad hoc committee said they'd reached consensus. I said, 'What's the difference between consensus and consent? I said I wouldn't sign.' The administrator said, 'Then you must move your wife to another hospital.' Our obstetrician objected because Karla was much too sick to move. The administrator said, 'If your child is born here and weighs more than 500 g, we will resuscitate it.'

"The administrator didn't bring me the written policies. And only in court [years later] did we find out that they had no policy. Their only policy was that, in the event of a conflict between doctors and parents, the hospital was required to get a court order to do what they wanted to do. But they never made that call during the eleven hours that they had between the time of my refusal to sign and the time of Sidney's birth.

"By mid-afternoon, they asked me for my insurance card for 'supplemental insurance.' Karla and I worked at the same place, but they re-papered the forms because my card had twice the insurance coverage that Karla's card had."

At 11:03 p.m., the "tragic miscarriage" ended, and Sidney Miller was born. She weighed 1 pound and 5.6 ounces and was "limp and blue," according to court documents. Mark said that she could fit in the palm of his hand. Her hand, when splayed out, was the size of his thumbnail, and her head was somewhere between the sizes of a golf ball and a tennis ball. Her eyes were fused shut.

The Millers expected the delivery room staff to wipe the vernix—the "cheesy varnish" that covers fetuses—off the baby, diaper her, swaddle her in a blanket, and hand her to her parents. But instead, a young neonatologist who had been sent into the delivery room by the hospital's administrator and whom the Millers had never seen before immediately "bagged" and "intubated" the baby and connected her to a ventilator. Mark said that the ventilator was one designed for adults and that it had no settings for such a preterm infant.

"They overrode my express refusal," Mark said, "and they didn't go get a judge. They had time to change the insurance papers, but they didn't have time to find a judge. There is a judge in Houston twenty-four hours a day who waits at a telephone to rule on these decisions. The administrator was playing God, not knowing that role had already been filled. A nurse who saw what had gone on in the delivery room said to me, 'get a lawyer.'"

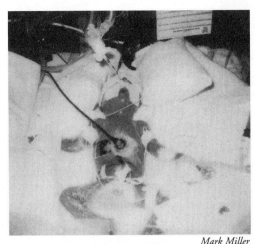

Mark Miller
Sidney intubated and connected to a ventilator

The baby immediately became the victim of aggressive intensive care. Her spine was tapped; she received blood transfusions and intravenous injections.

"They blew out every artery and vein in her arms and legs," Mark said. "They eventually put a central line in her chest so they could take blood and inject drugs. They routinely drained fluid from her brain by sticking a hypodermic needle into her fontanelle. They said, 'we are going to force oxygen into her lungs to keep her alive.' Then they said, 'a child this young doesn't have lungs.' Call it what you want. I'm calling it experimentation. But I did *not* give them permission to experiment on my child."

On the second day of Sidney's life, her brain began to bleed.

In the ensuing weeks and months, Sidney stayed on a fast-moving treatment train.

"I signed every consent form they gave me after she was born whenever they proved one of three things to me," Mark said, "that the intervention would prevent further damage to her body, that it would alleviate her pain, or that it would move her toward a better quality of life. Signing consents for those purposes is an easy choice, something every parent can understand. But this was very different from our refusal before her birth to sign a form to let them experiment."

Sidney spent close to eight months in NICUs at the Woman's Hospital of Texas and, later, at Texas Children's Hospital, where neurosurgeons tried seven times to place a shunt in her brain to drain away the fluids that were collecting there. When she finally went home, her care required round-the-clock nurses for several months. By then, the Millers' one-million-dollar insurance policy had been completely depleted.

"There is a motive for a for-profit health care giant to choose and make decisions for aggressive treatments," Mark said. "When Sidney was in the NICU, everything was on bar codes. If they used a syringe, they recorded the bar code on Sidney's chart. I saw them bring barcodes from stuff they used on indigent children and put it on Sidney's chart. We got charged $35 for a circumcision tray. I'm gonna go out on a limb and say I'm pretty sure my daughter didn't get a circumcision."

The Millers sued the Woman's Hospital of Texas and its parent company, Columbia/Hospital Corporation of America, for negligence and battery and for performing experimental treatments on their baby without their consent. They didn't sue the resident who had resuscitated the baby or any of the other doctors. In explaining that decision to me, Mark said, "Our lawyers wanted us to sue the doctors, but it was the hospital administrators who made the decisions for our child. They made them over our objections. There were clearly defined procedures—like getting a court order—that would have precluded and remedied any differences we had, but they didn't seek them. HCA picked my daughter's care. But she wasn't their child, she wasn't the child of a Board member, and she wasn't an indigent child. They depleted our one-million-dollar policy and walked away from their decisions, which sentenced our daughter to the life she lives today.

"I wasn't prepared to blame doctors. They did what they were told by the hospital. My problem is that my house has mirrors. I don't feel comfortable looking at the mirror every morning and saying, 'I ruined someone's career.' This trial was not about money. No amount of money on this earth is going to fix Sidney's many maladies or return Karla's life to her."

At the trial (January 1998), the Millers' lawyers pointed out that, at birth, Sidney was premature, but she was not disabled. She was turned into a severely disabled person by the many interventions imposed on her by the hospital.

"My child had no handicaps when she was born," Mark told me. "All her handicaps were the results of a treatment alternative chosen by a hospital administrator. Who has the right to make healthcare decisions for your children? Unless you prove you are stupid, drunk, have no sense, you have the

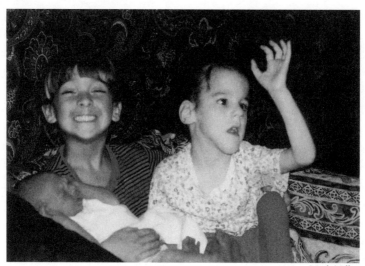

Mark Miller

Sidney with her younger brothers

right to make these choices. They took that right away from us. This is not a triangle. This is a straight line: doctor on one end, my wife on the other. Hospital administrator is not in there. I'm real sure of that."

At the time the case came to trial, Sidney was seven years old. She was legally blind, severely mentally retarded, had cerebral palsy, had seizures, could not feed herself, could not sit up, walk, talk, or be toilet trained. The shunt was still draining fluids from her brain, and she still needed—and would always need—round-the-clock care.

The trial lasted two weeks. The Texas jury of six women and six men found the hospital grossly negligent in its treatment of Sidney and in its blatant disregard for her parents' clearly articulated advance directive, which was to provide only comfort care to their fetal infant, even though that probably meant that she would die soon after her birth. The jury found that Sidney was born prematurely, that she was not born disabled, and that her disabilities were caused by the actions of doctors acting as the agents of the hospital.

The jury awarded the Millers $29,400,000 in damages for Sidney's lifelong medical expenses, $17,503,066 in accrued interest on these expenses, and $13,500,000 as a punishment. The punitive award was a notice to HCA and to other hospitals that parents' wishes are to be honored and upheld.

As part of his testimony in court defending his actions to resuscitate Sidney, the resident said, "In general, all babies are normal children or fairly normal children," an odd comment considering that Sidney was a 22- to 23-week fetus.

The Millers did not bring Sidney to the courthouse during the trial. "We didn't want pity or sympathy," Mark said. "HCA threatened to subpoena Sidney. They said they didn't want any shenanigans from us—they didn't want us to bring her down on the final day so that the jury would stare at her and not listen to their arguments. But the trial was not about pity. It was about who is going to care for Sidney when I can't."

When the trial ended, the members of the jury asked the Millers to stick around to talk. Two jurors who had voted against the settlement said that they had cast 'no' votes only because they felt the award was not large enough. Mark asked one juror when it was that he made up his mind about the case. The juror said, "Day one. I looked at your table. You had one lawyer. I looked at their table. They had twelve lawyers in blue suits. And I thought, 'They must have screwed up, and they must have screwed up big to need so many lawyers.'"

The huge award was an unmistakable message from the jury that in their judgment a colossal injustice had been done to the Miller family by the agents and administrators of the hospital.

The story had a biblical quality—a first-born child, administrators playing God, the victory of an individual over a (corporate) giant.

But three years later (December 28, 2000), the metaphor collapsed. The goliath hospital corporation appealed to the Court of Appeals for the Fourteenth Circuit of Texas. And, in a 2:1 decision, the judges reversed the jury's decision. The Millers were to "take nothing" for Sidney's lifelong care.

The two judges who ruled against the Millers said that Texas law *did* give parents the right to consent to medical care for their children and to withhold treatments. And the hospital *was* required to get a court order when there is a dispute between parents and doctors. But for each of these stipulations, the judges had discovered a caveat.

First, withholding treatments: this was only allowed if the child's condition was certifiably terminal; the judges found it impossible to know if Sidney's condition was terminal until she was born.

As for the court order: the requirement did not hold in emergency situations. They found Sidney's condition to be urgent, "emergent," at her birth, and this exonerated the doctors from their actions, even though those actions were in opposition to the parents' expressed wishes; the judges used the emergency exemption to exonerate the hospital as well from failing to get a court order.

The dissenting judge didn't buy his colleagues' arguments. He wrote that the hospital *did* need a court order to overrule the parents because that would provide "an impartial tribunal" for determining whether the fetal infant's best interests would be served by resuscitation and aggressive intensive care or by being allowed to die.

In addition, he found that there had been no emergency because the parents had stated their preferences eleven hours before Sidney was born.

"A true medical emergency," he wrote, "is where a doctor must operate and no one is available to give the proper consent. The Millers were present in the hospital at all times leading up to the birth and resuscitation, but [the hospital] chose not to try to change the Millers' minds, change doctors, or try to obtain a court order. Anytime a group of doctors and a hospital administration has the luxury of multiple meetings to change the original doctors' medical opinions . . . there is no medical emergency."

The Millers appealed the appellate court's ruling in the Texas Supreme Court, where oral arguments were heard on April 3, 2002. The supreme court justices hammered away at the hospital's attorneys, asking more than once what authority the hospital thought it had to override the parents' wishes and restating the jury's conclusion that battery had been committed on Sidney when the delivery room doctors acted without the Millers' consent and against their wishes.

Thus, it was a total surprise when, a year and one-half after the oral arguments, the Texas Supreme Court affirmed the ruling of the appellate court (September 30, 2003).

I called the dissenting justice from the appellate court, Maurice Amidei, to ask him about the appellate court and supreme court decisions.

"I thought it was a cockeyed decision," Justice Amidei said about the appellate court's majority decision, "not based on either the pleadings or the facts of the case.

"On the appellate court, we don't know the people, and we don't get emotionally involved. We don't see parties or witnesses. All the lying has already been done by the witnesses, the lawyers, and others.

"We have to stick to the facts and to the law. We have to look at the written record. I looked and looked and looked. I couldn't find where one witness testified or where in the written pleadings anyone said that it was an emergency. So, if no one alleged it or proved it, it can't be in the case. A conservative judge is one who makes decisions by applying laws and facts. If that had been done for the Miller case, the appellate court would have upheld the jury decision. They dreamed up this 'emergency' concept. It came out of the sky somewhere."

Why did he think the Texas Supreme Court affirmed the appellate court's decision?

"In ninety percent of cases where the Texas Supreme Court grants a writ of review," Justice Amidei said, "it's because they will reverse a decision or do something drastic, like change an award. The Texas Supreme Court grants a review to only about one in forty cases. And they don't grant reviews just to bring in the attorneys and tell them how good they are!

"I think that if the supreme court had decided it right away, the decision would have been different. But by the time they signed off on it, the members of the court were new. And that's a shame.

"I heard various justices say that they thought it was a hard case, the most difficult case they had. I didn't think it was a hard case. I was very disappointed in how it came out. Not all cases are decided correctly. Judges are human; sometimes they miss the boat."

I also asked Mark Miller about the discrepancies between the Texas Supreme Court justices' oral arguments and their written decision. He said, "It took eighteen months for the hospital to get the thing bought off."

The Millers' story has been discussed widely in the ethics, legal, and medical literatures and in professional seminars. In "Bad Cases Make Bad Law," two lawyers, one a theologian, comment that in the absence of "indications of neglect or malevolence, decisions for extremely premature newborns whose course is uncertain or ambiguous should continue to reside with those who bear responsibility for the infant—the parents."[1]

---

[1] John J. Paris and Frank Reardon, "Bad Cases Make Bad Law: HCA v. Miller Is Not a Guide for Resuscitation of Extremely Premature Newborns," *Journal of Perinatology*, 2001, 21: 541–544.

Bill Silverman commented on what happened to the Millers. "How, in the name of common decency, can rescuers justify their decision, free of all personal risk, when they override parents' refusal? They are allowed to walk away scot-free . . . [yet their] action results in the devastation of a young family. [They] are not required to pay one cent of the crushing lifetime financial cost, nor do they bear the family's tremendous emotional burden [for an] infant surviving with severe damage."[2]

Many newspapers and magazines have published feature stories about Sidney. After the trial, but before the decision was overturned, CBS's *Sixty Minutes* did a segment about the family. On that program, a Memphis obstetrician who was not involved with the Millers said, "If the baby is viable, I will resuscitate." The host, Lesley Stahl, pressed him: "You talk about saving babies. Saving them for what? . . . Just to breathe? Why should you decide instead of the mother and father?"

"No administrator at any for-profit hospital should ever be allowed to have a voice in the decision-making process that sentences a child to the life my daughter now lives," Mark said. "This court chose to rewrite one hundred and fifty years of Texas law. They took facts that were never brought before the jury or argued as a defense. They used them to spin an opinion that allows the corporation and its doctors to avoid responsibility for their negligence and actions and protects them from liability. When you hear on the news about 'judicial activism' and how the citizens need to be aware of judges writing legislation from the bench, here is an example of that practice."

LAW VERSUS ETHICS

Whenever a decision relating to medical ethics ends up in the courts it's a bad sign. The dilemmas that arise in NICUs are about individuals' lives—the lives of babies, the lives of parents. The courts turn these intensely personal struggles into dispassionate legal disputes and sometimes appalling public spectacles.

---

[2] William A. Silverman, "Mandatory Rescue of Fetal Infants," *Paediatric and Perinatal Epidemiology*, 2005, 19(2): 86–87.

The real issues—the quality of a baby's life and the life of a family—get lost in the chaos of verbal jousting. And, as Mark Miller said, precedents get set that can affect the lives of all babies born in the future.

Aggressive overtreatments of critically ill babies and those born at the margins of life, like Sidney, were widespread in NICUs in the United States beginning in the mid-1980s.

The technological imperative was strong and growing.

Intensivists were curious about pushing the margin of viability to earlier and earlier gestation times, often with little regard for the nature and quality of the long-term outcomes for the baby and the family—those whom *When Miracle Baby Grows Up* refers to as "Cinderella children."

Parents were clamoring for miracles.

And, as Gary Horn mentioned, fear and paranoia about undertreatment of sick babies were pervasive because of the Baby Doe regulations. One estimate by health professionals who work with disabled children is that 250,000 disabled babies, who would have died, were kept alive because of this fear and paranoia during the height of the Baby Doe era.

BABY DOE

"Baby Doe" was born in Bloomington, Indiana, on April 9, 1982. He was a full-term baby, the third child of his thirty-one-year-old mother. He was born with genetic and visible physical anomalies—Down syndrome, an enlarged heart, and an esophagus that ended in a blind pouch.

The baby was limp and blue at birth; he was having a hard time breathing. The obstetrician advised the parents that, even though a surgeon could fix the baby's esophagus, the quality of the baby's life might be poor and the cost of raising him might reach one million dollars.

The father, a school teacher who had worked with some children with Down syndrome, also was concerned that his son's life might end up being of "minimally acceptable quality." Baby Doe's parents decided not to allow the surgeons to operate on their son, and six days later the baby died.

But during those six days, a number of people who were not directly associated with the family—administrators at the hospital, some pediatricians, and right-to-life activists—challenged the parents' decision not to authorize surgery. They convened a late-night hearing at the hospital with a judge from the county. They asked the judge to force the parents to have the esophageal fistula repaired. But the judge was unwilling to rule against the parents' right to make decisions for their own baby.

Then the county's district attorney stepped in, but higher courts—the circuit court of the county and, later, Indiana's supreme court—also sided with the parents. At that point, the group appealed to the U.S. Supreme Court, asking for an emergency ruling to force the parents to accept surgery, but that's when the baby died.

The death of Baby Doe did not, however, end the wrangling.

The incident interested President Reagan and Everett Koop, his surgeon general, because both of them were strongly opposed to abortion and to the concept of letting sick and severely impaired newborns die peacefully. Reagan assigned to the Justice Department and the Department of Health and Human Services the task of finding a legal mechanism for forcing resuscitations and other treatments on all future newborns, no matter how sick or impaired they were at birth.

The federal authorities sent a poster to every NICU in the United States. The poster had to be displayed on the NICU's outside wall:

> DISCRIMINATORY FAILURE TO FEED AND
> CARE FOR HANDICAPPED INFANTS IN THIS
> FACILITY IS PROHIBITED BY FEDERAL LAW.

Should anyone suspect that a sick baby was being denied aggressive interventions, that person was instructed to call a hotline and report the possible violation; the hotline's 800 number was posted next to the sign.

The government convened "Baby Doe Squads" of lawyers, hospital administrators, and doctors. These people stood poised to fly anywhere in the country to investigate suspected violations of the Baby Doe regulations. One hospital that was investigated by a Baby Doe squad characterized the squad's methods as "a blitzkrieg by the Baby Doe Gestapo." The squad breezed into town, raced to the hospital, swooped down on the NICU, and seized the baby's chart.

Individual pediatricians and eventually the American Academy of Pediatrics vehemently objected to the squads and their methods. And after eighteen months, their objections and the bad press that the squads were receiving halted the squads' activities. More than 1,600 calls had come into the hotline, and the federal government had investigated forty-nine of them, but they found no violations of federal laws.

The Baby Doe rules proved unenforceable, but the paranoid climate that they engendered lingered. And the rules remain on the books.[3]

One bioethicist who surveyed physicians in perinatal medicine in the late 1980s reported that two thirds of these pediatricians felt that the Baby Doe regulations "interfered with the parents' right to determine what course of action was in the best interests of their children," that 60 percent believed that "the regulations did not allow adequate consideration of infants' suffering," and that 32 percent said that "maximal life-prolonging treatment was not in the best interests of babies but that the Baby Doe regulations required such treatment."

The bioethicist noted that the Baby Doe regulations singled out infants "for a set of rules that most adults would not tolerate for themselves." A heartless double standard was victimizing the voiceless newborns. "Adults, facing a choice between prolonging life and preventing a life of minimal or no consciousness or of pain and suffering," she wrote, "sometimes believe that there are worse things than dying.

"If we agree that it is wrong to do to others what we would not want for ourselves," she added, then the Baby Doe regulations had to be discarded.[4]

A comment in "The Principles for Family-Centered Neonatal Care" captures the irony of the Baby Doe regulations:

"It is a cruel paradox that this law, intended to protect infants from neglectful undertreatment, now promotes abusive overtreatment."

SEVE

"Seve was rescued by doctors who were caught in a Baby Doe mentality," Kathryn Neale Manalo told me. Kathryn's son Seve was seventeen years old when we spoke.

---

[3] Gregory Pence, *Classic Cases in Medical Ethics*, New York: McGraw-Hill, 4th ed., 2004.

[4] Loretta M. Kopelman, "Are the 21-Year-Old Baby Doe Rules Misunderstood or Mistaken?" *Pediatrics*, 2005, 115: 797–802. Loretta M. Kopelman, Thomas G. Irons, Arthur E. Kopelman, "Neonatologists Judge the 'Baby Doe' Regulations," New *England Journal of Medicine*, 1988, 318(11): 677–683.

"I call Seve's birth my 'aborted miscarriage.' Part of our family lore was the story of how my mother lost her second pregnancy," Kathryn said. "My mother had dropped twenty-five pounds during her pregnancy, and her obstetrician knew that she would lose her baby. It happened while she was at the beauty parlor.

"The day that I woke up in wet sheets feeling crampy, I called the obstetrics clinic for advice. I took my older son to school. I broke into tears in the car while I was driving myself to the clinic. It was then the realization hit me: Oh, gosh. Another second-pregnancy miscarriage, just like my mom's. When I got to the clinic, I said to the staff, 'I'm in labor and I'm having a miscarriage. And I don't want to scare all these pregnant women.'"

But unbeknownst to her, Kathryn had just walked into a Baby Doe-fearing hospital, and that meant that Seve received both immediate and continuing aggressive interventions in the NICU. Kathryn described a litany of procedures that Seve endured over many months and years, including early encounters with an eye doctor who, she'd been warned, "finishes the eye exam even if a child is coding."

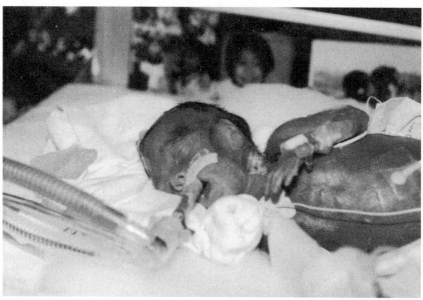

Kathryn Neale Manalo

Seve at one month

"There is nothing instinctual about putting a tube down the throat of your child to feed him," Kathryn said. "I had held and breast fed my first son. But Seve was completely resistant to being held. I hardly felt like his mother. I think he hated being held because he was tortured in some way every time someone picked him up. I felt that all the things that were done to him—the tube down his throat and so on—were abusive, and I began to feel complicit in the abuse."

Outsiders did not disabuse Kathryn of that perception.

"The first time I took Seve to the supermarket," Kathryn said, "he stopped breathing. I began to do the chest percussion I'd been taught for un-clogging his airways, and someone came up and said to me, 'stop beating your baby or I'll call the police.'"

The state of California pays for appropriate care, and thus when Kathryn and her husband finally took their baby home, they had state-supported nurses helping them for one shift a day—except on weekends—for the next two years.

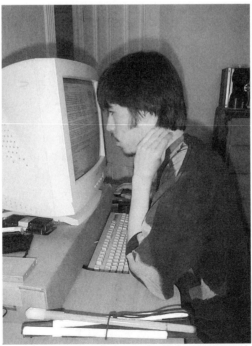

Kathryn Neale Manalo
Seve reading the computer screen

Kathryn was attending the 2005 Hot Topics meeting when she and I met. She was there to talk to intensivists about aggressive interventions from the parent's perspective (still raw after seventeen years), about her insights on outcomes (still unfolding with her son), and about the threat that she perceived from the Born Alive Infants Protection Act (BAIPA), which the U.S. Congress passed in 2002. She worried that this new Act could restore to NICUs the Baby Doe paranoia of the 1980s and 1990s. In fact, she said, it would actually make Baby Doe look like a walk in the park.

"BABY DOE REDUX"

BAIPA was approved by both houses of Congress with little fanfare. Even the Neonatal Resuscitation Steering Committee of the American Academy of Pediatrics gave it an easy pass, concluding that BAIPA would not affect standard delivery room decision-making practices.

But a 2005 critique of BAIPA by neonatologist-lawyer Sadath Sayeed—titled "Baby Doe Redux?"—shows that BAIPA has the potential to permit "jurisdictional creep" of federal officials and equally dangerous intrusions by "prudent layperson observers" back into the NICU.[5] Their demands could, with BAIPA backing, intimidate intensivists, overturn reasonable obstetrics practices, and interfere with the choices of parents, much as the Baby Doe regulations had done.

Sayeed's critique was prompted by an announcement in April 2005 by the Secretary of the Department of Health and Human Services that his agency would "investigate all circumstances where individuals and entities are reported to be withholding medical care from an infant born alive. . . ." The Act was to apply to "every infant member of the species *Homo sapiens* who is born alive at any stage of development."

What concerned Sayeed was that BAIPA acknowledged no generally agreed-upon procedures, such as those suggested by the American Academy of Pediatrics, for handling babies who are born at the margins of viability. BAIPA also failed to consider the best interests of babies and the interests of

---

[5] Sadath A. Sayeed, "Baby Doe Redux?" *Pediatrics*, 2005, 116(4): 576–585.

their families, and it made no mention of the likely quality of life of saved or salvaged babies.

Sayeed cited the Millers' lawsuit, noting how "judicial decisions undermine the ethical discretion that parents are typically afforded in decision making before and after delivery in these morally complex situations."

"The implementation of this new directive," wrote Sayeed, "suggests an intrusive future in which governmental oversight of treatment decisions involving imperiled newborns returns to hospital obstetric and nursery suites." And, as has been clear from all of the past experiences with the Baby Doe regulations, the squads, the many lawsuits between parents and physicians and hospitals, "the law and its supporting regulations remain a clumsy vehicle for controlling bedside decision making for the imperiled newborn."

CONNECTING THE DOTS

"I am wondering who it is who is legislating this life for these extreme preemies," Kathryn said to me, "and who is planning to pay for them.

"What are we doing when we insist that parents take this on? When a woman gets pregnant, does she automatically give up her rights to life, liberty, and the pursuit of happiness? What is the reason that our society is insisting on all of this suffering?

"I've been wondering also why child abuse is seen only as neglect and not also as putting babies through these tortures. Exactly whose interests are being served by these experiments on preemies?"

The day the BAIPA regulations were approved, California announced a state-wide reduction in in-home services for disabled residents. Kathryn had been struck by the juxtaposition.

"When you save a baby in the NICU," Kathryn said, "there is a ripple effect—medical expenses, educational expenses. Who will bear the financial burdens and the life consequences for these decisions? Here in California, universal preschool will be on the ballot, and people are arguing that it will cost too much. How does the insistence that we resuscitate babies and then educate them in special schools fit in here? Is the distinction that there's no profit in education, but there is profit in medical technologies?"

Chapter 11

Money Matters

The first time I heard the term "profit center" in connection with the NICU was when I asked Bill Silverman to explain to me why some micropreemies had been so aggressively overtreated.

"Follow the money," he said.

Would a NICU really seek to make a profit at the expense of an innocent baby and the family?

Some parents I spoke with—Gary Horn, Mark Miller, and others—were certain that their newborns had been singled out for saving or salvaging precisely because they, the future parents, had arrived at the hospital with lucrative insurance packages.

And soon articles and editorials began appearing in the medical and ethics literatures explaining how NICUs had become "the profit centers" and "the economic engines" of certain children's hospitals and general hospitals. Without their NICUs, many hospitals would actually have to fold.

What was especially unsettling to Bill was the possibility that individual doctors sometimes have the option to become shareholders in the hospitals where they work. He pointed me, for example, to a website where neonatologists are encouraged to join a giant international neonatal healthcare enterprise. When a doctor's income is tied directly to the profits of the hospital, he said, surely there would be times when the interests of the baby and the doctor's own financial interests might not be exactly congruent and the doctor might place financial concerns first.

Doctors who would do this would, of course, be violating their core vow to do no harm.

One modern version of the Hippocratic oath expresses the doctors' avowed commitments this way: "I swear to fulfill, to the best of my ability and judgment, this covenant: . . . I will apply, for the benefit of the sick, all measures that are required, avoiding those twin traps of overtreatment and therapeutic nihilism . . . I must not play at God . . . I will remember that I do not treat a fever chart . . . but a sick human being, whose illness may affect the person's family and economic stability. My responsibility includes these related problems, if I am to care adequately for the sick . . . I remain a member of society, with special obligations to all my fellow human beings, those sound of mind and body as well as the infirm . . . May I always act so as to preserve the finest traditions of my calling . . . healing those who seek my help."[1]

Those are the commitments that doctors make. But in an avaricious era, such as ours, only the naïve would hold that there never will be a doctor who might be seduced away from the profession's intrinsic virtues by economic enticements. The hope, of course, is that only rarely would a doctor do this.

I had a conversation not long ago with a doctor—but not a NICU doctor—who said he had been "dueling on the chart" with his partner about what to do for a dying patient. The partner was ordering one more procedure—billable at many hundreds of dollars—that both of them knew was futile for the patient who was very close to death. The doctor I spoke with was upset that his partner was so mercenary, so enamored of the economic benefits of ordering expensive, futile medical procedures.

EVOLUTION OF PEDIATRICS

That some NICUs have become profit centers seems to have been an inadvertent development along with shifts in the focus of the field of pediatrics. One hundred years ago, pediatrics did not even exist. Then, at the 1912 Iowa

---

[1] http://www.pbs.org/wgbh/nova/doctors/oath_modern.html

State Fair, the president of the Iowa Congress of Mothers posed this question: "If a hog is worth saving, why not a baby?"

That question triggered action. At the next fair, a team of tent-based physicians stood ready to evaluate local babies, much as judges in a nearby tent were evaluating the hogs.

"If there is a standard for calves and colts," noted the popular magazine *Outlook* in 1913, "why not for babies, in order that each mother may strive toward that standard for her child."

The Iowa State Fair and other fairs across the country touted the accomplishments of the people who lived in the local communities—the flowers they raised, the cattle and hogs they bred—and thus it was also natural for them to look closely at the condition of the local human "stock."

The tent-based judging soon evolved into Better Baby Contests. My own mother was evaluated in one of those contests when she was thirty-nine months old. Bill Silverman told me that his baby brother had also been a contestant in a Better Baby Contest, that one in Southern California.

Each baby was scrutinized for specific physical characteristics and graded for various developmental and behavioral criteria. My mother's score card was filled out by four different examiners in Middlesboro, Kentucky—J.P. Edmond, L.L. Robertson, W.F. Marx, and L. Wilson.

Robertson docked her ten points for "weak feet" and another ten for "knock knees," Edmond and Marx registered no complaints, and Wilson just recorded her height (thirty-seven inches), her weight (thirty-one pounds), and her sleeping habits (with her mother, with one window open). I am guessing that the form they filled out—published and distributed by the Better Baby's Bureau of the Woman's Home Companion in New York—was the same form that the California judges used to rate Bill's brother.

These Better Baby Contests became controversial. Parents were not pleased to be told that their babies did not measure up. Nevertheless, they evolved into something constructive—rudimentary well-baby clinics. Doctors began attending to babies not only at fairs and not only when the babies were sick but also when the babies were well. The doctors developed expertise in child development and soon could give parents guidance on how to promote their babies' health. The specialty of pediatrics had taken root.

Through the first half of the twentieth century, many harrowing and sometimes deadly childhood illnesses required lengthy hospitalizations, and

Better Babies
Standard Score Card

Entry No. _93_ Division _7th._
Score_____ Age in Months _____
Rural_____ City_____
Male_____ Female_____
Name _Layette Helen Heinlein_
City and State _Middlesboro Ky_
Street and Number _116 Chester Ave_
Weight at birth_____ lbs.
Strong or weak at birth _Strong_
1st, 2d, 3d, 4th, 5th, 6th, 7th, 8th, 9th, 10th child _6th_
Breast-fed _Yes_ No. months _3 ms_
Mixed-fed (bottle and breast)_____
No. months_____
Bottle-fed _____ How many months _____
What foods_____
Amount of milk in each feeding_____
Number of feedings now in 24 hours_____
Kind of food at present_____
Sleeps alone_____
If not, with whom _Mother_
Sleeps in open air_____
Windows open _Yes_ How many _1_
Father's name_____
Age _45_ Nationality_____
Occupation _Contractor_
Mother's maiden name_____
Age_____ Nationality_____
Occupation _Housekeeper_
Has birth been registered_____
Where _Middlesboro Ky_
Contest held at _Middlesboro Ky_
By _Red Cross_
Date _May 1 - 22_

ISSUED BY THE
BETTER BABIES BUREAU
WOMAN'S HOME COMPANION
381 Fourth Avenue, New York
Copyright, 1913, 1914, by The Crowell Publishing Company

See important note on the last page of the card

A page from the author's mother's Better Babies Standard Score Card pediatric wings expanded in general hospitals to accommodate all of the sick children. Later, whole hospitals were constructed that were dedicated solely to the care of children.

With the mid-century development of vaccines, a number of the brutal childhood illnesses—polio is a prime example of this—were beaten back. And along with the discovery and development of antibiotic therapies, the common epidemic infectious diseases of childhood increasingly could be treated on an outpatient basis.

Thus, by the final quarter of the twentieth century, the need for pediatric beds in hospitals began to shrink. Just one pediatric subspecialty was burgeoning—neonatal intensive care. And it was proving to be the "economic lifeblood" of pediatrics and sometimes even the hospital.

EPIDEMIC OF PREMATURITY

The raging pediatric "epidemic" then became, and still is today, the epidemic of prematurity. Older women trying to have babies late in life began increasingly to resort to fertility drugs and other reproductive technologies. These interventions increase the likelihood that twins, triplets, or higher multiples will be born, and most multiples are born prematurely. At the other extreme of the mothers' age spectrum are very young women, who frequently have their babies early, especially if they have neglected their bodies, care little about nutrition, and have not sought prenatal care. Drug addicts, ever increasing in numbers, commonly give birth early. And finally, a subset of women began electing to have their babies delivered through Caesarean sections before they reached full term for their own or their doctors' scheduling convenience.

"We imagine that we are working to protect premature babies because they need us," wrote a pediatrician/bioethicist in 2001, "but it turns out that preemies are also working for us. They perform an important altruistic function for our medical centers.

"Pediatrics departments and children's hospitals are now financially dependent on NICU preemies. Over the past three years, [my] NICU has had the highest revenue-to-expense ratio of any unit in the entire hospital, including both adult and pediatric units. Recognizing this fact, [my institution's] new Children's Hospital, like most new children's hospitals, will have more NICU beds than the current one but will not have room left over for a new emergency department, new outpatient clinics, or an auditorium for public gatherings."

The community's endorsement of the concept of the NICU shows, he wrote, that NICUs "make a compelling moral claim upon society. This claim insists that we not turn our back on these tiny, vulnerable babies. . . . NICUs [are] the epitome of our humanity, the measure of our devotion, the test of our will. NICUs stand for our society's moral commitment to children . . . recognizing that our tiniest citizens have rights."[2]

---

[2] John D. Lantos, "Hooked on Neonatology," *Health Affairs*, 2001, 20(5): 233–240.

Chapter 12

Experimenting with Babies

Exactly what rights are communities granting newborns? And what about protections?

When, for example, politicians or judges or hospital owners and administrators impose Baby Doe regulations or BAIPA-style requirements on micropreemies and other fragile babies, the resulting life and suffering of the child and the family get disregarded in favor of political, social, or economic agendas. Their perspectives are cruel and myopic: the insistence on rescue is rarely backed by an equal insistence on ensuring that the children and the families receive long-term support.

The doctors in the television documentary *When Miracle Baby Grows Up* and many parents and intensivists have spoken out about the enormous suffering of babies who received excessive or medically inappropriate treatments. Can better protections be put in place to shield future babies from also becoming "experimental animals?" Clearly, when neonatologists experiment on babies, the goal must be to ensure that most of them end up as lucky ducks, not drubbed human guinea pigs.

ETHICAL PROTECTIONS

The boundary can often be blurry between an actual experiment—called a clinical trial—and a standard clinical treatment. When, in 1979, the U.S. National Commission for the Protection of Human Subjects of Biomedical and Behavioral Research published federal guidelines for protecting individuals who participate in clinical trials, the report included an important cautionary note: distinguishing medical experimentation from medical practice is, at times, almost impossible. This certainly holds true for babies, whose bodies are so vulnerable and function in such primal fashion.

The quintessential ethical requirements that this commission's *Belmont Report* identified for clinical experiments—and which are also relevant to medical practice—are these:

- The reason to carry out any test of a new therapy, drug, or other intervention must be to eventually do some good.
- Those who are asked to take the most risks must also be those who will be the first to benefit, should the findings prove useful. That is, benefits and burdens must be distributed fairly. Drugs and treatments cannot be tested, for example, only on poor babies and then be used only for the benefit of rich ones.
- The wishes and preferences of the participants—or, in the case of babies, their parents or other proxy decision makers—must be respected.

These three requirements are rooted in three of the key principles of medical ethics—beneficence, justice, and autonomy.

How respect for parental autonomy—the third requirement—is realized is through the complicated process of getting informed consent before any experiment on a baby begins.

Getting informed consent is tricky at all times, and getting it in the NICU is no exception. The setting is tense, sometimes rushed, and usually emotionally charged. Parents may be so desperate to try anything—the therapeutic imperative—and so anxious as their baby hovers between life and death, that they may not actually hear how risky, how uncertain, or even how experimental a drug or procedure or other intervention is. In addition, parents are never tested to make sure that they fully and accurately understand what they were told. Thus, consent is often not *truly* informed.

Parents may agree to interventions for their babies without grasping that the intervention is only experimental, not an established treatment. This phenomenon—the therapeutic misconception—is well known in all clinical settings, not just in the NICU. As Brian Carter pointed out, all treatments are interventions but not all interventions are treatments. Parents who fall into this trap, this misconception, sometimes expect much more from an intervention than it could ever be expected to deliver.

The guidelines in the *Belmont Report* apply specifically to clinical research that is funded by the federal government. They are not enforceable for trials run by pharmaceutical companies, and they do not strictly relate to standard medical care. Still, the spirit of the guidelines—with their calls for respecting parental autonomy, beneficent behavior by doctors, and the fair distribution of treatments—underlies what is appropriate for all trials, no matter who funds them, and for all medical care as well.

A pediatrician-bioethicist noted in a 2004 editorial that, because federal regulations make it extremely difficult to enroll babies in clinical trials, a great deal of the clinical innovation in the NICU today is happening outside formal research protocols.

"This leads to increased risk for patients," he wrote, "and it decreases the quality of the knowledge gained by such innovation."[1]

"PREEMIES ON STEROIDS"

An example of how a breach in the research-treatment boundary resulted in grim, adverse effects on babies came to light in 2000, when researchers reported that steroids, widely used in the 1980s and 1990s in perinatal medicine, had caused numerous long-term harms and even short-term problems that had not previously been documented. This disaster was serious in the way that the oxygen blindness of the 1950s was.

Certain steroids were known to promote fetal lung development. So pregnant women who were at risk for early deliveries began receiving a course of steroids, and when their babies were born, the babies also received them.

---

[1] John D. Lantos, "Pediatric Research: What Is Broken and What Needs to Be Fixed," *Journal of Pediatrics*, 2004, 144: 147–149.

The steroids worked well, giving the babies' lungs just the boost they needed to cope with their early exposure to air.

But sometimes one of these women did not, after all, go into early labor. If she stayed pregnant for a few more weeks, she might then receive a second course of steroids. These additional doses of steroids were given without any careful demonstration that they produced additional benefits. The outcome studies suggested that they might even be causing harm.

Steroids were also given to babies who could not easily be extubated. When such babies received steroids, they could be freed from their ventilators within forty-eight hours. But fifteen years later, follow-up studies showed that the babies who received steroids for this problem had high incidences of neurological deficits and cerebral palsy.

The discovery of these long-term and some new short-term effects (hypertension, infections) shocked the medical community. One group of California doctors wrote that they had been "seduced by the siren song of postnatal steroids," and they called for a moratorium on steroid use: "It is now time to reconsider and curtail our current clinical practices," they wrote, "until such time as appropriate studies demonstrate acceptable short-term and long-term benefit without unacceptable harm . . . Only clinical trials that meet these minimal criteria should receive institutional review board approval and local and national funding."[2]

On reflection, no one should have been so surprised that powerful agents, like steroids, would affect not just the specific lung cells that they were meant to target but also other cells throughout the babies' bodies. Steroids are not magic bullets but broad-spectrum biochemicals; and all cells of a baby are sensitive to outside influences because they are in such a rapid phase of differentiation, development, and growth.

Helen Harrison learned about the problems with steroids at the 2000 Hot Topics meeting. She passed the information along to parents of preemies and a year later published a paper in the journal *Birth* titled "Preemies on Steroids: A New Iatrogenic Disaster?"

Parents, she wrote, had not been told "of the known and suspected risks of multiple prenatal or postnatal steroids. A few parents [said] they were told

---

[2] Neil Finer et al, "Postnatal Steroids: Short-term Gain, Long-term Pain?" *Journal of Pediatrics*, 2000, 137(1): 9–13.

the drugs might 'slow growth,' but complications involving the brain, eyes, and other organs and systems were never mentioned . . . [Parents were] angry that they were never given this information . . . [They were] devastated to discover that many of the illnesses and disabilities their children now suffer may have resulted from, or been complicated by, the use of steroids."

A neonatologist, commenting on the Internet, found it odd that "as physicians, we get informed consent for standard procedures with clear risk-benefit balance, such as immunizations and blood transfusions, yet are not necessarily expected to get consent for postnatal corticosteroids where there is no standard for use, and significant potential for harm."

"The time has come," Helen concluded, "for parents, who with their children must live with the outcomes, and for the public, who ultimately pay for this care and its consequences, to be honestly informed about the 'experimental' nature of neonatal treatment for very preterm infants and its unfortunate results. It is also time for parents and the public to demand that steroids and, in fact, all poorly evaluated neonatal treatments be used only in the context of formal clinical trials."

INNOVATION DILEMMA

I went to talk to Siva about the steroid fiasco. How, actually, does one safely try new therapeutic strategies that might help babies? In effect, is it ever possible not to experiment? I wanted to discuss with him the blurry boundary between clinical research and standard clinical practices. I could see how the tug of the therapeutic imperative could be, at once, compelling and problematic for everyone concerned.

"We have to be careful," Siva said. "We need to use our intellects and our wisdom when we innovate. But we don't have the license to try whatever we want."

Many problems, he said, stand in the way of introducing new procedures and new drugs into the NICU.

When, for example, a drug like a steroid has been shown in a clinical trial to be effective for one indication or for one type of baby, the drug manufacturers tend to be reluctant to fund further clinical trials to test that same drug on another category of babies or for related but not identical problems. Do

I do nothing or do I try to adapt that drug to situations that are related to the situation in which I know the drug is effective?

The postnatal steroids, for example, had worked beautifully in getting babies extubated. And there was preliminary information, from one randomized study and anecdotally, that they produced short-term benefits.

But this points to another obvious and perpetual dilemma, Siva said: you can't know the long-term effects in the short term.

"We keep looking for better biological and chemical markers that will correlate with long-term effects," he said. The developmental delays and cerebral palsy associated with steroids took about eight or ten years to begin showing up. If the babies had not received the steroids, they probably would have died. But they stayed alive, and only later did their problems appear.

APNEA OF PREMATURITY

Siva then told me about another common problem—apnea of prematurity— that he felt illustrated in a very visual way how treatment strategies can evolve outside clinical trials. Apnea is easily observed—the baby stops breathing— and many of the early interventions were low tech.

First came the physical and mechanical approaches. In the 1960s, intensivists would tie a long string around a baby's foot and thread the free end of the string to the outside of the incubator. The nurses would pull on the strings often, to jostle the babies. They hoped this would keep the babies from falling into such deep sleeps that they would fail to breathe. (Having the strings outside the incubators meant that the incubator's controlled environmental conditions did not need to be disrupted every time the string was pulled.)

In the 1970s, babies with apnea were placed on waterbeds. The idea here was that the undulating bed might keep the babies somewhat stimulated. But the waterbeds got messy, especially in a setting where so many needles were in use.

Next came the biochemical approaches. The asthma drug theophylline was a bronchodilator and it might help to stimulate breathing. But theophylline produced some bad side effects—reflux, too rapid a heart rate.

What about caffeine, the stimulant that was keeping the babies' parents awake? Caffeine proved to be much safer than any other compound in a series of small, controlled clinical trials, and it had more therapeutic latitude. Today it is used for many babies who have apnea episodes.

Chapter 13

Desirable Outcomes

"Siva," I said. "Do you *truly* believe that a 26-week preemie can ever do well? Wouldn't it just make better sense to stop experimenting with early preemies and establish a surer, later, cut-off point for rescuing preemies so that there would be less suffering?"

We had talked often about the uncertainty of outcomes, and Siva had been the first doctor to tell me about the importance of involving parents in the NICU's difficult decision-making processes. I knew that he knew about bad outcomes. Now I, too, knew about them first hand from a number of the parents I had met.

Siva's response was immediate, and it was confident: his NICU really did have many examples of babies who were born that early, had been followed closely, and had done well.

As if on cue, the intercom buzzed on Siva's desk. His department's administrative officer asked if he could take a minute to step outside; the twins had arrived, and they wanted to see him. Siva turned to me and laughed. "Come meet these kids," he said. "They were born at 26 weeks."

MEREDITH AND BENNY

I expected to see infants or maybe a set of toddlers in the anteroom. But standing there were the nineteen-year-old twins, Meredith and Benjamin, and their mother Lynn Kriss. Every year since the twins' birth, Lynn had either brought her children up to the NICU on their birthday or had sent in a cake for the staff.

Everyone hugged Siva and a second doctor who had been pivotal to the twins' survival two decades earlier. What a reunion! Everyone was smiling; everyone was excited.

When the kissing stopped, the conversation focused first on Benny who, everyone agreed, had entered the world with an enormous will to live.

Benny had not been expected to survive. But according to Siva, Benny's intrepid personality had been obvious at his birth. He was a born fighter, evidenced by the fact that by the end of his first day of life he had pulled out all of his IV lines.

The NICU nurses had nicknamed Benny "The Linebacker," and they had posted a sign with that moniker on his incubator. Someone speculated that this sign must have had a subliminal influence on Benny because in high school he had, in fact, been his football team's linebacker.

Then everyone turned to Meredith and began asking her about her interest in going to nursing school. Meredith had started to think about becoming a nurse—probably a NICU nurse—after her last visit to the NICU. (The family had lived away from Washington for a number of years, and they had skipped some of their birthday visits, but four years earlier they had stopped by on their birthday.) Meredith had been deeply touched by the nurses she saw on that last visit, how they had remembered her struggles during the weeks she was in the NICU, and how they had cried from happiness to see that she had grown up healthy.

Benny pulled up his shirt and turned to Siva.

"Tell me what this scar is. How about this one? What about this?" And Siva, like a guide at some tourist attraction, explained the provenance of each of the scars on Benny's back and belly. Then Siva asked Benny how the scar was on his forehead, and Benny swept his wavy hair aside to show Siva that NICU battle wound.

Meredith and Benny were charming. They were in town on their winter break; both are first-year college students. Their exquisitely timed visit to the NICU proved to me, as Siva had said, that sometimes a 26 weeker—in fact, two of them—could do very well.

NICU LEGACIES

Lynn Kriss had seven miscarriages between the birth of her first-born son and her pregnancy with the twins. So as a precaution, her obstetrician prescribed bed rest long before the twin pregnancy had even reached the halfway mark. Her doctor hoped this would protect the twins from the risks that are associated with developing inside an incompetent uterus made even more perilous by a total placenta previa.

Lynn's husband Lenny had taken their six-year-old son Michael to an ice hockey game when Lynn was 20-weeks pregnant, and he and Michael had returned home to find Lynn in crisis. Blood was flowing out of Lynn "as fast as water coming out of a sink that is turned on high." Lenny sent Michael across the street to get the neighbor, a physician. "Mommy's bleeding, mommy's bleeding," Michael yelled. "Come quick."

Lenny and their neighbor packed Lynn and stacks of beach towels into the car and raced to the hospital. Lynn was still conscious when they got to the hospital, and she vividly recalls the feeling of the transfused blood coursing through her empty arteries and veins.

During the next six weeks, Lynn received eleven more transfusions to replace the huge blood clots "the size of shoes" that streamed out of her body.

The twins managed to stay inside and develop until the 26th week of gestation, despite all of the physiological chaos and the massive blood losses that Lynn was experiencing. Siva and the other NICU doctors regularly visited her to talk about their plans for caring for the babies in the NICU once they were born.

That happened on January 5, 1987.

The doctors thought that Meredith—who was more robust at two pounds—had a good chance of surviving, but that Benny—at one pound and four ounces—did not.

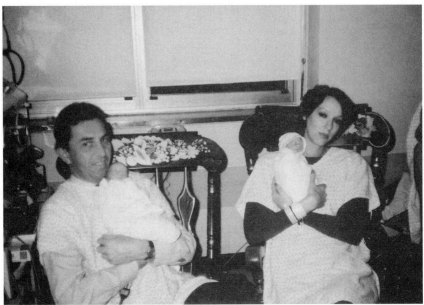

Meredith and Benny in the Georgetown nursery; their parents are holding them.

Lynn left the hospital five days after the twins were born, but she took no babies with her. She said that leaving them behind that day marked that as the worst day of her life.

About five weeks later, around Valentine's Day, Meredith went home, and a month after that so did Benny. Both babies were on monitors, both had oxygen, and Benny's first year was filled with trauma. He vomited constantly, had serious viral infections that required rehospitalization, and required nursing care around the clock.

The day that Meredith went home, Lynn insisted on taking a family photograph in the NICU. She persuaded the NICU staff to disconnect Benny from all of the tubes and monitors, so that he would look less fragile in the family photo. This picture is in their album, and once, when the twins were little and Meredith was looking at the picture, she said, "How come Benny is blue, Mommy?"

Benny told me that he feels extraordinarily close to Siva and the other NICU doctors and nurses. "We must have formed a relationship," Benny said, "but of course I don't actually remember them. I only now understand

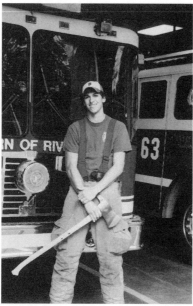

Lynn Kriss

Benny doing what he loves

what they did for me, and I owe them so much. I think it's not a fluke that I feel they are my best friends. When I talk to Siva I think 'this guy was in my life when I was a baby.'"

Benny also has long felt a strong pull to emergency situations. In high school he volunteered with the local fire department, now he is an EMT, and he might end up being an ER doctor.

"I'd probably be a fireman if financial stability were not an issue," he said. "It's heroic and it's extremely difficult."

Does all of this relate to his early time in the NICU?

"I don't remember the NICU," he said, "but perhaps I remember the spirit."

(A mother of another preemie told me that her son's closest relationship today is with his computer. She said that, when the hard drive on his computer was crashing, he was overwrought. He came to her and said that he knew it was totally irrational to be so upset but he just couldn't help it. "He acted as though his life depended on a computer monitor," his mother said, "which, at one time, it did.")

The twins' NICU experience didn't just influence their trajectories but also that of their older brother. Michael told me about "standing on tippy toes" to look in at his siblings the day after they were born.

"When I looked the first time," Michael said, "I thought 'that doesn't even look like a person.' I also thought 'why does it take so many people to take care of them?'"

Michael said he went from "being an only child, getting everything I wanted" to being in a situation where the twins needed attention from "mom, dad, me, and ten other people! This helped me develop an intense awareness of other people and what they were going through, rather than just being interested in what was happening to me. I often felt, growing up, that I owed someone something for having my brother and sister."

Michael was impressed by the doctors who cared for the babies, and he was aware of their devotion to their work. "They were always at the hospital, always taking care of my brother and sister, always responsible for their lives." Their absolute commitment was what inspired him to go to medical school, where he is now.

"It's amazing, really a miracle, when you see those babies," Benny said. "Maybe once or twice a year I wake up and say, 'I was a preemie.' I was so lucky. Sometimes I think 'if I could overcome that, I can overcome anything.'"

Chapter 14

Life in the NICU

I wanted to spend more time in the NICU. I wanted to see this environment more closely. I had gone on rounds with Siva and had toured other NICUs with other neonatologists. But now I wanted to see what a baby's day was like.

Siva suggested that I talk to Judy Diaz, a nurse who began working with him at Georgetown several decades earlier. She was there even before Benny and Meredith were infants and remembered them, although she wasn't directly involved with their care.

Judy invited me to shadow her on a day when she was working in the step-down feeder-grower nursery. That day, twelve babies were in the room, another sixteen were next door in the critical care nursery, and thirteen nurses were taking care of all of them.

Judy was caring for three babies and was expecting that a fourth one would move in from next door at any time. One of "her" three babies was a strong, beautiful boy who was not sick but just being observed because his mother had developed an infection right before she gave birth. The other two were sweet sisters, part of a threesome. Their "big" sister had already gone home. I appreciated anew the extent of human variability when I saw two newborns next to one another, one weighing four pounds and the other weighing eight.

Judy had already completed the head-to-toe assessments of the three babies in her charge by the time I got there—the check of their vital signs, the palpation of their bellies to make sure that they were soft, and so on. Every NICU shift begins that way.

The baby boy's mother and father were already in the NICU, and Judy was showing them a few basic things about how to care for their son. They both looked completely exhausted. Their baby was taking his time learning how to nurse, and he had not gotten anywhere near perfecting his technique.

Soon the mother got weepy—some combination of worry, frustration, fatigue, her infection. Judy turned to a technician and asked her to find out if the "Nesting Place" was available. When the technician returned and said that it was free, we walked the parents down the hall and showed them into the room—a typical hospital room with two beds—where they could take a nap. It was one of two such rooms; the other was called "Dad's Den," although it was for new mothers too.

Back in the NICU Judy focused her attention on the sisters. She fed the larger one a bottle.

The smaller one had been drinking from a bottle too, but she'd had too many "bradys" (episodes of bradycardia—drops in heart rate), and Judy was concerned that she might aspirate her food during the bottle-feeding. So Judy put six teaspoons of formula into a syringe, connected the end of the syringe to a tiny feeding tube that ran down the baby's esophagus and into her stomach—this is called gavage feeding—and then held onto the syringe as gravity took over the feeding of the baby. Judy kept checking to make sure that the flow was steady.

The father of the girls was now in the NICU. He and Judy were talking when the little one's monitor began to beep. Judy carefully suctioned the backed-up formula out of the baby's mouth and then readjusted the baby and her tubes.

The big girl was now about to face her "car-seat challenge." Could she sit in her car seat for an hour and maintain a stable heart rate and breathing? This was the day that she would be going home if everything checked out okay. The car seat was on the floor, and soon the baby was sitting in it.

All morning long, the nursery stayed busy, and the busy-ness was totally upbeat. One baby yowled intermittently whenever his pacifier fell out of his mouth; but as soon as someone reinserted it, he grew silent. An occupational therapist stopped at his crib and said to him, "You can scream that loud? It's time for you to go home!"

Parents were holding, rocking, and just staring at their babies. A mother of twins was off in a side isolation room with her children, one of whom had spiked a fever. But she seemed relaxed and smiled as I smiled at her.

Late in the morning, the boy's parents came back into the NICU. They were totally transformed.

"Thank you *so much* for getting the room for us, Judy," the mother said. It was clear that they had both taken serious naps, and they were now rested and eager to be with their son.

They checked his temperature, but it was too low for him to come out of his incubator. Judy thought that perhaps they had not positioned the thermometer in the right place, so a few minutes later, she told them to check his temperature again. This time it was fine. Judy checked his vital signs herself. "Perfect," she said, and out came the baby.

"Uh uh uh uh uh," the baby said, then he gurgled, and his mother whispered something to him. Judy set up a screen around the mother and baby to give them some privacy. But the baby was still not nursing, and after Judy suggested a few more things to try, she arranged for a lactation consultant to come up to the NICU to help the mother.

Around midday, the room got incredibly quiet. All of the babies had been fed, most were napping or rocking, and I got the impression that working in a NICU was not only wonderful fun but also totally routine, a piece of cake. Monitors were doing many of the tasks that nurses once did—checking heart rates, temperatures, the oxygenation of blood—and even gravity was doing some of the feeding. Judy had been filling out a lot of forms—too many! she said—but neither she nor any of the other nurses was breathless, harried, or dashing about.

At 1:50 p.m., the room actually became totally silent. Not a peep from anyone—baby or adult. Total peace. Judy told the other nurses that we were going out for lunch, and we left.

THE NICU TEAM

When we returned half an hour later—wow! Something was happening at every baby's station. A technician with a swooshing ultrasound machine was examining one baby's kidneys. The lactation consultant had brought up a new type of breast pump for the boy's mother to try and was giving her advice. A nurse and a mother were working with a baby who was having some trouble with reflux. A doctor was talking solicitously to a timid mother and was giving her reassuring pats on her arm. A social worker was on one of the telephones, arranging for some services. A doctor was on another telephone, ordering tests. The triplets' mother had come in with the biggest of the trio, and now all three sisters were there with both of their parents. So much for serenity; the place was abuzz.

Siva had often told me about the "team" approach of the NICU. And here were many of the team members in action. These little babies and their parents were being scrutinized and helped by not just nurses and doctors but also a range of specialized therapists (speech, occupational, lactation, others) social workers, psychologists, pharmacologists, nutritionists, people from the pastoral care department.

Several people had gathered around the triplets and their parents. "We'll know that things are running smoothly at home if you come back to get the third one," one of the doctors said. Everyone laughed. "Actually," she added, "we should have a policy that, when you have multiples, we bring the last one to you!"

Judy chatted with the triplets' mother about what she anticipated for the smallest of the three babies and when she thought that baby might be ready to go home. She said she would coordinate the follow-up check-up for the second baby with the discharge of the third one, so that the parents wouldn't have to make a special trip to the hospital with the second baby.

Shortly after that, the triplets' parents headed home, this time taking with them two of their three newborn daughters. They seemed wistful about leaving the tiniest baby behind, but they were also philosophical.

CRITICAL CARE NURSERY

When we had a moment, Judy took me next door to look at the babies in critical care. The mood in that room was somber. None of the upbeat fun and none of the liveliness and hopefulness of the step-down nursery had carried over there. So many of the babies looked painfully fragile and vulnerable. Many were barely visible under layers of tape, monitor leads, and IV lines. Some were shockingly small. One baby's skin had an ashy tone. That baby had recently had intestinal surgery, and the edema had made her skin taut and accounted for its unnatural sheen.

We looked at a baby in a giraffe incubator; the incubator's cover could rise, making it easy for the nurses and doctors to reach in and minister to her. That baby was small, fetal. I could see why a baby like that might have a hard time ever catching up to a baby who was born at full term.

I thought about Sidney, Edward, David, Michael, Seve, Keegan, Holly, and their long weeks and months as preemies in NICUs.

I thought about how it had been NICU doctors who first suspected that Elly and Chloe might have genetic anomalies.

I realized that Clara and Benny and Meredith had all spent weeks in this very room when they were infants and had been so sick and needy.

Some babies *could* do well. But not all were lucky.

The nursery door swung open. In marched eight gowned, masked, and gloved escorts, bringing a baby back from surgery. They wheeled the baby's crib back to its place. Then the entourage of doctors, nurses, and technicians assembled around the baby's crib, watching for some time to make sure that the baby was stable.

In a corner of the room, close to the delivery suite, two stations were set up for assessing newly born babies. Everything was ready for the next baby— or two—who would show up.

NURSES AT THE CRIBSIDE

I had a chance to speak with several nurses that afternoon. Most estimated that they split their time almost fifty-fifty between working with the babies and working with the parents. One of the long-time nurses—one who had actually been involved in caring for Meredith and Benny—said that the NICU population had gotten heavily skewed toward preemies and away from sick babies in the years that she had been there. More than in the past, she said, mothers were having their children very late or very early in life.

"People say to me that it must be so sad to work in the NICU," another nurse said, "But it's mostly happy." She was a traveling nurse who worked for an agency that gave her twelve-week or fourteen-week assignments at different hospitals around the country. She was young, had no dependents, and so this was an ideal time for her to experience a variety of communities and work in different hospitals. She was just about to move on to a NICU in southern California.

"Particular babies you work with and care for can stay in your mind for a long time," Judy said. "Our hospital follows the families closely in the apnea and developmental clinics. So even after the babies leave the NICU, many of the parents come back to visit us after their appointments. It's wonderful because we can see how the babies are doing and how well the parents are coping.

"Every September, we have a NICU reunion that's just overwhelming. We have a moon bounce, balloons, face painting. So many parents and babies come back. They remember us. And it is so wonderful to see all of them and their progress. This year, one mother came whose baby died in the NICU. She wanted to see all of us.

"I think one of the special things about our unit is our dedication to families. We truly care for the mom and dad. Sometimes just sitting quietly at the bedside with the family is a great comfort to them. It especially helps them to have the same nurses taking care of their babies throughout their stays. This is called primary nursing, and it allows for continuity of care. It helps the family adjust better and become more comfortable asking questions and sharing their emotions.

"Trust is important in our relationship with the parents. They depend on our honesty and openness. We run support groups for the parents and grandparents twice a month to discuss a range of things, like how hard it is for them to leave the baby here at night and go home, how hard it is for them to leave the older siblings at home, how scary it is to come here. We also spend time teaching the parents how to talk to their babies, how to gently stimulate and touch them, how to give them skin-to-skin care—this is called kangaroo care. All of these things are great for bonding.

"Some days are quiet and uneventful in the NICU. These days we have down time. We keep the lights turned down, and we talk quietly. We spend extra time with the parents. But we always are prepared for a 'stat' buzzer from the delivery room or an urgent transport to bring a baby from another hospital.

"It's really amazing how well we all work together, especially when there's an emergency situation. We really enjoy working with each other, and that helps. Agency nurses comment on the special relationships we have here and so do parents who have had to take their children elsewhere—to other hospitals for special procedures—and then return. I think the parents see how well we work as a team, and they appreciate that."

Chapter 15

Death in the NICU

I asked the nurses then about the difficult days in the NICU and about the babies who are not likely to survive. One of the babies in the critical-care nursery was so critically ill, so physically deformed.

"Sometimes it cuts you in half," a nurse said, "seeing babies who are too small. It's hard because you never want to take away the parents' hopes. But when a baby weighs less than 500 grams, you *know* that child will never be right. How the attending physician presents information to the parents can really affect the decisions that the parents end up making. It's such a difficult time. But sometimes, even when the attendings present the information clearly, the parents just don't hear it. They are so engrossed in the moment.

"I'm a big patient advocate. When a baby is suffering, it can be so difficult. But when we have a situation like that, we call for an ethics consult. [The consult may involve one person or a committee, as explained in the preface.] There was a baby here recently, for example, who had little brain function. That baby was ready for palliative care. I always feel that, if palliative care is appropriate, we are ethically bound to offer it to the parents."

Her remarks reminded me of a longer conversation that I had with Chris Keller, a NICU nurse who works for a large midwestern hospital system. Chris splits her time between the high-end suburban NICU and the low-end downtown unit.

"I was the primary nurse some years ago for an infant with a genetic anomaly, called Trisomy 18," Chris told me. "The baby had a three-chambered heart, which is incompatible with life. She was on a ventilator. The mother was homeless, living in a shelter with her four-year-old son. She was angry with us, saying we were 'hounding' her to let us remove her baby from the ventilator. She grew angrier and angrier, complaining that we were saying all these things because the infant's care was costing the hospital money and she couldn't pay.

"I began by believing that the baby should be removed from the ventilator. An ethicist visited us from another hospital. And eventually the case went to the ethics board. But the mother was not invited; she wasn't even told about the consult. I thought this was wrong, so I went to the meeting, feeling it was my duty to represent the mother's point of view.

"I told the ethics board that the mother would eventually let us remove the baby from life support—but that she was asking for time to get to know her baby before the baby died. Those were the mother's words. She didn't care about longevity. She just wanted some more opportunities to see her baby's eyes and to see her lift her head just the slightest bit.

"Then I asked how much the cost of the baby's care was affecting the ethics decisions. The head of the committee was annoyed; he said that money had nothing to do with this.

"The committee eventually decided to ask the doctors not to harass the mother anymore about removing the baby from the ventilator. The medical director of the NICU decided to take over that case personally.

"Soon the mother was ready to let her baby be taken off the ventilator. A female bishop from the shelter came in to baptize the baby. The neonatologist removed the baby from the vent. The baby was in distress. The mother fled to the bathroom and locked herself in there. The neonatologist panicked, put the baby back on the vent momentarily, and then took her off again. So much drama!

"The mother then angrily refused the baptism. We found a rooming-in room for the mother, where she stayed with her baby for three days. The mother was very content—she held, fed, and slept with the baby. On the third morning, the mother found the baby dead in the bed. There was no drama at all.

"I had taken a picture of the baby late one night; I blew it up at Walgreen's on my way in and gave it to the mother when I came to be with her after the death. We washed and dressed the baby. There were many visitors, many tears, but mostly everything was peaceful. There was a great chaplain at the time, and we had a beautiful group prayer.

"When the baby died, we had been in the process of negotiating with the shelter to take the baby in with the mother and her four-year-old and to give them a private room, knowing that the baby was dying. It was the most amazing thing. I called and asked if the shelter would consider doing this, but I did not really expect them to say yes. But they did. It was a very open-minded and compassionate shelter.

"I changed lanes during that eight weeks with that baby. I started out believing, as my colleagues did, that removing life support was wise. But as the time went by, I saw the mother's position as valid. She needed to be ready. She needed time to say goodbye and to get to know her baby before she let her go. She needed some things to be in her control and on her own terms, rather than on the doctors' and nurses' terms. She got what she needed from us. Her baby had a peaceful death. I learned a ton. I changed the way I looked at things. I believe it was my best piece of work as a nurse."

ETHICAL BEHAVIOR

"I have other stories for you about ethics," Chris said.

A full-term baby "got into trouble" one night when Chris was working at the suburban NICU. The baby's father was watching anxiously as the neonatologist worked on the baby, trying to resuscitate him. At one point the father said, "Doc, if he is going to be messed up, you can stop right now." But the doctor didn't stop trying to resuscitate the baby nor did he say anything to the father.

"Why was there no chance for dialogue?" Chris asked. "What made that father say what he did? Was it appropriate for that neonatologist to completely blow the father off? The neonatologist didn't say what he was thinking, what he was doing, what his values were, what he is required to do legally or ethically, according to his Hippocratic oath. Why not, for Pete's sake???!!!"

(Siva has talked about four C's for ethical decision making—communication, clarification, consistency, and caring—all of which could have helped here.)

"I don't know if the dialogue ever got picked up later in the child's hospitalization," Chris continued. "I don't know if there was any discussion at the discharge rounds or during the care conferences about the potential consequences to this child of that aggressive resuscitation. To me, this was a case of a doctor with arrested ethical development."

But, Chris said, she had a third story that illustrated what she considered a really ethically sound decision. A nineteen-year-old woman came into the hospital in premature labor. She was 22 weeks and 6 days into her pregnancy. The fetus was in a breech presentation, and when the feet came out they were white and peely. For inexplicable reasons, the woman's cervix then snapped shut, and the baby's head got stuck inside for seventeen minutes.

"This baby did not have a snowball's chance to live," Chris said. "And when the baby finally came out, its neck was broken. Its eyes were fused, which means that the alveoli are not at the end of the bronchioles. You can't vent a baby that young, because there are no air sacs. The doctor heard heart tones, but he made the decision to wrap the baby in a blanket and hand the baby to the young mother. In ten minutes the baby died. It was merciful."

I heard a similar story about compassion and relieving a baby's suffering from a bioethicist who served on a pediatrics ethics committee at a Catholic facility. He said that the priests on the committee regularly insisted that the morally appropriate treatment for a seriously ill newborn was to withdraw aggressive life support. The priests cited Pope Pius XII's 1957 statement and the 1980 Vatican declaration that it was an "extraordinary, gravely burdensome, or disproportional treatment" to keep going with aggressive care. He recalled a devout Catholic couple who knew their tradition well and felt comfortable (from their religious perspective) when the time had come to let their baby die. Their decision to stop aggressive treatment was completely in accord with Vatican thinking, he said, yet was probably a violation of the Baby Doe rules.

VICTOR

My first contact with Chris Keller was not to talk about her experiences as a nurse, but because she sent me an intriguing email: "My adopted son, an ex-preemie, was a cocaine baby, one pound and six ounces, born in the toilet and left there."

Chris had not been working in the NICU the night the paramedics brought in the baby, Victor. No one knows how long he had been floating in the cold water of the toilet before someone saw him there and called 911. When the paramedics found Victor, his body temperature had dropped to eighty-nine degrees. His mother was an addict who had done crack cocaine five hours before his birth. He was born fifteen weeks before he should have been.

Victor's heart was barely beating, and only after four doses of epinephrine did the beat pick up; then the doctors connected him to a ventilator.

Victor had intractable seizures. Then serious brain bleeds. His head swelled as the blood clotted and blocked the flow of cerebrospinal fluid. The dammed-up fluids and the oxygen deficits were all wreaking havoc on his brain cells.

Neurosurgeons put a shunt into Victor's brain to drain the fluids, but the shunt didn't work. They tried a second time. Still no luck. Victor was labeled a "hopeless case."

The hospital contacted his birth mother, and she consented over the telephone to whatever the hospital wanted to do. The hospital decided to find a foster home where Victor could go, receive palliative care, and be allowed to die. By this time Victor was one hundred days old.

Chris had become Victor's primary nurse just two weeks before he was ready to leave the hospital. She had also just received a license to offer medical treatment foster care, and she decided that she would be the one who would take Victor home and care for him while he died.

Chris said that her decision to get a foster care license arose from the convergence of two experiences/ideas she had earlier in the year.

"I was tap dancing pretty fast to do my assignment one night," Chris said. Instead of the usual three babies that night, she was caring for four. Two of them were twins, and although they were not identical, Chris noticed that they were completely in synch with one another. Whenever she was ministering to one of them, the other baby seemed to know it: either both babies would calm down at once or, sometimes, when she fed one of them, the other one would wake right up and vie for her attention.

Chris began thinking what a shame it would be for the twins to be separated when they were placed in foster care. And then she began to wonder how the foster care placements actually were handled. So the next morning she called the Child Protective Services office and asked a social worker about the placement process.

The social worker said, "Why do you want to know? Would you take them?" That was a question that Chris had never considered before.

Shortly after that, around Thanksgiving, Chris was again working on the night shift in the downtown NICU's feeder-grower room. She was thinking about the nine babies who were there that night; none of them needed much medical attention, but none of them had any other place to go. Their mothers were all addicts, all were being treated for addictions, and all had lost custody of their babies. Chris knew that the nurses on duty that night really would have preferred to be at home with their families for the holiday. She fantasized how great it would be for the babies and the nurses if each nurse could take one baby home with her. (Her supervisor said, "Oh my God! The liability!")

It was then that Chris decided to become a medical treatment foster parent.

When the time came for Victor to leave the hospital, Chris lined up a pediatrician who was willing to care for a dying baby, and she arranged for hospice workers and nurses to come regularly to her home. Two of her own five biological children were available to help. What she expected was that Victor would not get better, only worse, and die.

"He was not a pretty sight," Chris said. "The shunt was still not working and his head kept growing. My fourteen-year-old was quite unnerved by his appearance—large, soft head and tiny preemie body.

"The IV feeding pump was in my kitchen. We fed him with a nasogastric tube. He slept most of the time. After five days in my home, though, the shunt just started working on its own. The big melon head decompressed abruptly, and a two-inch-deep furrow ran from Vic's forehead to the top of his head. His appearance was even more bizarre than it had been. I was shaken. The hospice nurses were taken aback."

But after about six weeks of expecting the baby to die, things changed.

"We were not just keeping him comfortable anymore," Chris said. "We began to shift our focus. What could we do to give him a more normal life? The hospice people stopped coming. And we started hoping.

"I thought I would have a baby for a short time," Chris said. But Victor thrived, and eventually Chris adopted him. He's "a wonderful feisty kid,"

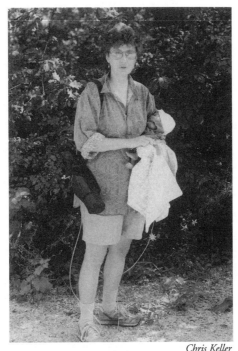

Chris Keller
Chris and Victor with oxygen tank and tubing

Chris said. But as is characteristic of so many other preemies, Victor's development fits no single category.

"Every child takes something from his NICU experience and carries it with him for the rest of his life," Chris said. "It could be a weakness in the respiratory system—lots of colds or even asthma later on. It could be neurological. It could be delayed development. Everyone has something.

"Vic is like other cocaine babies: as the years go by, they exhibit lots of attention deficit hyperactivity disorder symptoms. He never stops talking. He seems to understand things, but he may not be able to alter his behavior. His hearing is super-acute. He has the vocabulary of a college freshman, he has perfect diction, and he will remember multisyllabic words forever.

"But he does not know how to chew or swallow food, he walks on his toes, he has quite a few of these autistic features, but he doesn't have that diagnosis. He has memorized about eighty picture books; he reads like a first grader (he's in fifth grade). He has no depth perception, and he doesn't gather information with his eyes. His eyes are structurally sound, but his visual cortex—the picture screen in his brain—is what's problematic. Still, he is proficient at shooting baskets, and he'll make three or four holes-in-one in a game of miniature golf.

"Vic blew us away by achieving his gold belt in Tae Kwon Do. I really thought he'd never learn his 'form,' which requires right-left moves and one hundred and eighty degree turns. He doesn't know left from right. In any case, he did it.

"We used to take him to lots of plays, but now sometimes he's inappropriate. It's not cute when a boy his size talks during a performance. I have to rush him out of these places.

"We all have turning-point moments that we remember in our child's life—those moments when we realized what the score was going to be. These are not the same moments as when we first heard the hints, facts, initial diagnoses, or prognoses. For parents of preemies, they are often memorable for

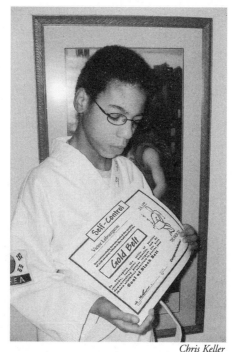

Chris Keller
Vic with his Tae Kwon Do Gold Belt award

the distress they cause. The individualized educational plan meetings, one each year at least, that take away your breath and your equilibrium and your hope all at once—and you are supposed to be a strong advocate for your child while you are brought to your knees! The day they test your child's IQ and the number is below eighty. Vic's IQ is forty-eight, and his mental age is between two and a half and four years.

"I had a long period of coming to accept Vic's IQ. And this makes me realize that if even I could not accept what Victor's IQ of forty-eight implied, why do I expect young parents I meet in the NICU to accept the truth about their babies? Most of the young mothers just don't seem to be as interested in outcomes as they should be. But I also see that the truth hurts too much. It takes time to accept.

"I've had to finally accept that my child will never be independent. And I'm terrified about that. I never envisioned that I'd have a teenager when I was in my sixties."

Chapter 16

Immense Suffering

This concern—who will care for my needy child when I cannot?—haunts so many parents I have met.

Some hope or expect that their other children will care for the child who is dependent when they no longer can. Many talked about how limited services are now for children and adults with special needs and how, rather than expanding programs, governments and communities are cutting them.

One of the parents I met and first interviewed some years ago has special expertise in the area of disabilities. Jack Schutzius works at the Service Employees International Union, and he had, by chance, been assigned to work with direct-care workers—those who support people with disabilities—about a year before his son Brian was born with a serious chromosome anomaly.

Jack knows many adults who have disabilities. He told me that the quality of life for many of them was much better than he had expected, even though they were experiencing pain and had many obvious difficulties. But, Jack said, "Their lives would be better if they weren't so poorly supported."

Recently he told me that, in New Orleans, after hurricane Katrina, 22 percent of the people who remained behind did so because they were disabled, and an equal number of people stayed there in order to care for their disabled relatives and friends.

"The disabled," Jack said, "are poor, invisible, and powerless. Even when disabled kids have huge entitlement, the moment they hit eighteen, they get nothing."

BRIAN

I had connected with Jack and his wife Laura Fries in 2002. One of my students at Johns Hopkins University stopped me after a class and said that her sister's baby was having problems and that her sister—Laura—wanted to talk to someone.

I wasn't clear exactly how I fit in—I was writing about babies, not providing care for them. But by then, I knew many doctors and researchers, and I had spoken to many parents who were grappling with difficult challenges with their sick children. I thought that perhaps I could help Laura connect with resources or people who might help her.

I went to Laura's and Jack's home in Virginia. Their son Brian was eighteen months old at the time. He was lying on a blanket in the living room, and he slept through most of the two-hour conversation that Laura and I had.

Brian's lovely soft skin was ivory colored. His face was incredibly sweet. He didn't move too much, but I wasn't sure how much of his immobility had to do with the fact that his right leg was encased in an ankle-to-knee cast. Perhaps the cast was acting as an anchor.

Laura had been suspicious during her pregnancy that something might be wrong with the baby. And she even worried that the problem might reside in the baby's genes because she and her sister-in-law had both had problems associated with childbirth. Laura had a miscarriage two years earlier, and Jack's sister had given birth to a boy who lived only eight days, and she too had recently had a miscarriage. No one had, though, identified a specific genetic anomaly in the family.

Laura said that when Brian was born the doctor announced, "It's a big, beautiful boy." But those had been the "two seconds of joy" that she and Jack had at the birth of their son, because the doctor quickly added, "Oh, but he does have a clubfoot."

The staff whisked Brian to a corner of the delivery room for his newborn work-up, and Laura said she was able to watch from the delivery table as the

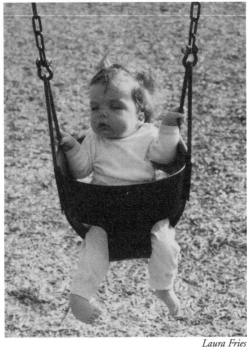

Laura Fries

Brian at six months

nurses and doctors examined Brian. His Apgar score—an assessment of the baby's color, heart rate, muscle tone, and reflexes—was good: eight on a ten-point scale. But at one moment, a nurse took her eyes off Brian and glanced over toward Laura, and that's when Laura knew that more bad news was to follow.

"The baby has a cataract, clubfeet, intestinal problems, a ventricular septal defect," the pediatrician casually rattled off. This news, both on its own and coming after what had happened to Jack's sister's baby, was desolating.

Brian was transferred to the NICU of a nearby hospital, where he stayed for seven weeks. He battled infections, fatigue, severe reflux, and other problems. He had transfusions, stomach surgery, X-rays, CT scans, light therapy, and countless other tests and procedures. When he finally left the hospital, he still had many problems, but he seemed to be growing and developing.

By the time Brian was six months old, he could sit up, hold up his head, and make good eye contact with his right eye; his left eye was blind.

Laura showed me a picture of Brian when he was six months old. He was sitting in a swing. His cheeks were chubby. His blond hair was rumpled and blowing in the breeze. He was holding on to the swing's struts, and only the curve of his foot suggested that anything might be amiss. A typical, engaging six-month-old.

But right after that picture was taken, Brian began to have seizures. For the next year and one-half, Brian had hundreds of seizures a day.

Often infantile spasms will subside as a child grows older. But Brian's did not. For eighteen months, the seizures were unrelenting, and none of the standard epilepsy drugs—Topamax, Klonopin, Keppra, Lamictal, Lorazepam—could control them. On good days Brian might escape with just a few seizures. But more typically he would be rocked by sixty to one hundred seizures a day. Such an intense level of seismic activity clearly was jarring to his body and impeding the growth and development of his brain.

The geneticists took about a year to identify the genetic basis for Brian's physical and metabolic problems. Some genes were missing from one of his #11 chromosomes, and in their place were genes from a #12 chromosome. Brian's #12 chromosomes were unaltered. The extra genes, or the missing ones, or both, probably accounted for Brian's enigmatic physiology. Such an anomaly is known as an unbalanced translocation.

The geneticists collected cell samples from many members of Laura's and Jack's families. Jack, his brother, and his sister all had balanced genetic translocations in the region where Brian's unbalanced translocation was. In Jack's generation, chromosome #11 had genes from chromosome #12 and vice versa. The complete, though rearranged, complement of genes kept Jack and his siblings from suffering from the problems that Brian had.

The hospitals where Laura and her sister-in-law had their miscarriages and where her sister-in-law's baby had died had stored samples of tissues from those three boys. The geneticists discovered that all three had the same unbalanced translocation that Brian had.

"Obviously this is a fatal genetic problem," Laura said to me. "There were three little boys in our family who didn't make it. Brian did. He's a survivor."

A genetics researcher I spoke to told me that "gene dosage" problems like Brian's—too many copies of a gene or too few—can sometimes tip the balance toward disease or dysfunction in ways that a few anomalous genes will not. But at this stage in our understanding of human chromosomes and the human genome, he said, there is no way to treat individuals for most chromosome anomalies—translocations, inactive genes, deletions, duplications, mutations—because "the damage is already done."

Brian was a survivor, but he continued to struggle. Several months before his second birthday, he was re-evaluated at the epilepsy clinic at Children's Hospital in Washington. The technicians hooked twenty-eight electrodes to his body and videotaped him for twenty-four hours. They wanted to see if his brain was developing, and they wanted to try to figure out where his seizures were coming from. Might there be new treatment options for him?

Laura stayed with Brian all day in the hospital, and Jack stayed all night. They were asked to write down everything that happened—when the seizures occurred, what happened, what each seizure was like.

Some weeks later, Laura and Jack returned to the clinic to discuss the findings. The news was not encouraging. Brian's brain was not functioning any better than it had a year earlier. It was growing, but only slowly, and some of the structures in his brain were atypical. The one hundred seizures that occurred during that twenty-four-hour period were originating in his brain stem. This meant that Brian was not a candidate for brain surgery. And although some new drugs were on the market, they were associated with fatal rashes, vision losses, and other unacceptable side effects.

Laura said that she came away from that consult thinking, "We have reached a gambling point. We have to take some risks."

She had read about a diet that helped some people whose seizures, like Brian's, were unresponsive to other treatments. A clinic at Johns Hopkins Hospital had pioneered this "ketogenic diet," which Laura said was "like Atkins, only more so."

The idea for the diet sprang from a faith healer/osteopath's observations early in the twentieth century that children who had been experiencing unremitting seizures stopped seizing after days of fasting and prayer. Scientists took a closer look at how such a diet might work. They found that, when the body's cells are deprived of sugar as an energy source, they break down fats into products called ketones. But exactly how ketone metabolism halted seizures is still not known.

The focus of the ketogenic diet is fat. Whipping cream, butter, eggs, oil, bacon, and cheese are the staples. For babies, like Brian, the fat comes in a "keto formula."

In 1997, Meryl Streep played the role of a mother in the movie *First Do No Harm*, which is based on the true story of a boy—Charlie—who, like Brian, had unremitting epileptic seizures. Charlie's father is a Hollywood director, and Streep knew the family. Many of the bit parts in the film are played by people who had epilepsy but stopped seizing when they went on the diet. The person who plays the Johns Hopkins dietician in the movie is actually the hospital's dietician; she had, by then, worked for more than forty years developing the diet and helping families adapt it for their relatives who suffer from epilepsy.

When I saw *First Do No Harm* and read about Charlie and his truly miraculous freedom from unrelenting seizures, I felt hopeful for the first time that perhaps Brian's future, too, could be a good one. The profile of Charlie— not the Charlie of the movie but the real Charlie—seemed almost exactly like Brian.

At Brian's second birthday party, which was also his big sister Emma's sixth birthday party, Laura and Jack were excited. Brian was old enough and big enough to try the ketogenic diet, and he was going to check into Johns Hopkins Hospital on April 1 to begin the regimen.

Two weeks after Brian started on the diet his seizures dropped from one hundred a day to about four.

"We're very excited," Laura said when I spoke to her then. "But we know it's not a miracle cure. He seems different. He's making eye contact. He's rubbing his eyes. He's sleeping through the night. He's cooing again. The yelling is gone. He was on pause for a year and a half. If the diet really does take away the seizures, then we can ask, 'Who is he and where do we go from here?'"

With the seizures greatly reduced, Brian began attending a school for children with special needs. Laura said she kept thinking that, if he could do things once—before he began having seizures—then surely he would eventually get back the skills and abilities that he once had.

But Brian's progress was not linear, and only in the fourth year of his life did he begin to regain some of the simple responses, like smiling, that he had been capable of as an infant.

I called Laura in early November 2005 to set up a time when she and Brian and I could get together again. I wanted to see how Brian was growing and catch up on the family. We decided to meet on November 15 at her house. In our brief phone conversation, she said that Brian was really doing great, and that, at a doctor's appointment the previous week, the doctor had been impressed with his recent progress.

So I was stunned when Laura's sister called me on November 10 to tell me that Brian was critically ill in the hospital and that she was not even sure he was going to survive. Here was a child who had endured so many trials and crises; surely this was just another one of them.

But it was not. On November 13, Brian died. His brain swelled, his brain stem shut down, he had a stroke, and his heart stopped beating. Doctors and nurses from all over the hospital raced to his room when the public address system announced the "code blue." Laura and Jack stood there watching for forty-five minutes as the staff tried to resuscitate Brian.

Finally Laura said, "Just stop."

The doctor who was coordinating the effort looked at her and said, "You've made the right choice."

A few months after Brian's death, Laura and I met for lunch. It was not hard to talk about what a tender little boy he was, but it was incredibly sad.

"The minute he was born, he had the sweetest, most knowing look," Laura said. "My mother thought that he would have had the same personality even if he had been born healthy."

I had talked to Laura's mother when Brian was younger. She told me then that, when she first saw him in the hospital in his crib, he was so beautiful that he had immediately captured her heart. She was just hopeful that he would be able to develop and be free from pain; she hoped he knew he was loved and would feel secure. She said she knew that Brian had a rough road to travel and "we have no road map for this; we don't even know where we are going."

I had also talked to Jack's mother. She said she hoped for a few miracles— that the seizures would stop, that he would have a chance to develop, that he would not be too damaged by his genes and the seizures. "He is my grandson and I love him," she said. She had intense anxiety about his future because she felt that the United States was unwilling to embrace the kinds of social programs that Brian would need as he grew.

Brian was not just prized by his relatives but also affected the thinking of people who barely knew him.

"Brian set standards," Laura said, "and people who met him will never look at disabled children again in quite the same way. That's a triumph. What was remarkable was what he did with what he had."

Laura mentioned a woman who had visited Brian's school to consider sending her daughter—who had autism—there.

"She said that I seemed to be treating Brian like a 'piece of gold,'" Laura said, "and she later told me that she thought to herself, 'If that woman can treat her son with such pride, I can learn to feel that way too about my child.'"

When the *Washington Post* published an article that I wrote about Brian shortly after he started on the ketogenic diet—this was when he was doing well—I received mail and email from a number of *Post* readers.

One woman wrote me that "I had a difficult time getting to sleep the first two nights after reading about Brian, thinking about the pain that this little child has had to endure so early in life. I was wondering if there is anything I can do for this family . . ."

I sent the letter on to Laura and Jack, who also had been getting feedback about the article. Laura sent the woman a note, and later the woman wrote to me again, this time in appreciation: "Laura wrote me a wonderful note at Christmas enclosing a beautiful small photo of Brian. It sits framed in green matting on the third shelf of my bookcase—and always will. If I can do nothing else for Brian at this time, I can (and do) think of him and pray for him."

"Brian made us look at life differently," Laura said. "Parents of severely disabled children are not part of the mainstream. Society shoved us into another room. Brian opened doors and we saw the world differently, and that has enriched our lives."

I had lunch with Jack recently. He was carrying Brian's picture in his pocket and grieving deeply for his son. As time had gone by, Jack said his hopes for Brian's future had been fading. Brian had not been growing, he had not been gaining much weight, and he was not developing. And although his son had been somewhat more engaged—he was responding when he was tickled and he was smiling more often—Jack felt that Brian's future might be impossible.

"It was challenging," Jack said, "to think about living a whole life with such limited capacity. It would have been challenging, too, for us, had he survived, but I wish he had."

ISOLATION

Laura once said that the experience of having a child with serious disabilities had made her feel like the character Gulliver in Jonathan Swift's classic book *Gulliver's Travels*. When Gulliver returned to his home from his years of travel, he no longer felt at ease with the life he previously had lived. He could not dismiss what he had learned or return simply to the old ways. He had seen other worlds, other beings, and other styles of existence.

Laura had said then, "It's been a strange odyssey, being in the subculture of sick children. Every negative thing that happens is like an arrow through your heart. And now that we've taken this journey, we can't go back.

"We've learned that having healthy children is such a gift. If Brian had been healthy, we probably still would not know that, still not have a clue. And that seems shameful to me now."

BUBBLE BOY

The isolation and ostracization that Laura described reminded me of the boy in the bubble, David. Was David's plight an apt metaphor for how our society treats the families of sick children—sealing them inside solitary social bubbles and leaving them to fight for survival?

I had followed the bubble boy's story as it was unfolding in the 1970s and 1980s because, as an immunologist, I was interested in David's disease— severe combined immune deficiency (SCID). But David's story was known well beyond immunology circles—and still is—because two movies depicted (and greatly trivialized) his experience.

At the time that David was born in 1971, his parents had already endured the death of a baby son from SCID. They spoke with doctors at Texas Children's Hospital and Baylor College of Medicine to discuss the odds of their having another baby with the same devastating condition. The amniocentesis indicated that the developing fetus was male and thus had a 50 percent chance of having SCID. But the doctors were optimistic that a cure for SCID was right around the corner. They encouraged David's mother to go forward with her pregnancy, which she did.

The hospital built a sterile environment in which David could be isolated immediately upon his birth. That way, he would not encounter infectious agents, which, because of his immunologic deficiencies, would quickly kill him. David did have SCID, and he was placed immediately in the bubble. But the doctors turned out to be woefully wrong about the cure-around-the-corner, and David lived in isolation for twelve years. Then he died.

A pastoral counselor at the hospital where David lived and died wrote of his profound discomfort with David's "rescue" and with those who had considered it appropriate to subject David, a human being, to such an inhumane life. A spokesperson for the medical team had outraged him by saying that "David's life has been important for medicine but his greatest contribution was his death, because with this information we will be able to treat other children yet to be born." (The spokesperson was wrong. SCID is still a fatal disease.)

"Technology and scientific knowledge are only pieces of the whole human experience," wrote the pastor, "but the medical establishment seems to act as if they are the whole . . . If we do not attempt to clarify soon what makes human life human, we may see even more monstrous dehumanizations than those experienced by David."[1]

THE NICU BUBBLE

I had been guided to that pastor's article by philosopher Andy Jameton, whom I met at a bioethics meeting in late 2005. Andy had written an eye-opening and iconoclastic article ten years earlier that had stayed in my mind ever since I first read it. His article was one of the few in the vast literature on NICUs that directly challenged their very existence and questioned their social value.

I asked Andy what had been in his mind when he wrote his article. He said he had been taken with the pastor's account of David's life in the bubble world and the island mentality that had shaped David's experience.

---

[1] Raymond Lawrence, "David the 'Bubble Boy' and the Boundaries of the Human," *Journal of the American Medical Association*, 1985, 253(1): 74–76.

Whereas I thought David's isolation was like that of the parents of sick children, Andy thought that David's life and the lives of babies in the NICU had many more parallels, both being so heavily steeped in mythologies about birth, life, rescues, and cures.

"The NICU represents an 'island mentality,'" he had written, "suggesting that economic development that improves the lives of a few people, while neglecting a vast peripheral population, is a sound strategy for coping with the global crisis of resources and population . . .

"The NICU must be a temporary historical phenomenon. Looking ahead fifty years to a world of a doubled population and even more greatly stressed world resources, it is incredible to think that we will continue to invest social resources in such an extravagant and unbalanced way; and, if we do, we may well be charged by the next generations with inhumanity . . . [as they] count the lives that were not saved because our culture neglected the larger picture of life and death."[2]

Andy said that now, a decade later, he no longer expects NICUs to vanish, in large measure because "profit centers are not very strict about whom they accept." He had, though, come to think more kindly about "rescue," although he felt that the U.S. investment in rescue, at the cost of public and environmental health, was still "majorly excessive."

But perhaps NICUs could make themselves more useful. They could be more discriminating. They could accept only babies whose chance for a healthy life was significant. They could stop accepting micropreemies and other babies who, in low-tech settings, would simply die—the ones who Bill Silverman had told me were once labeled stillborn. They could stop accepting babies whose "cures" were still just fantasies around the same elusive corner where the cure for SCID apparently still hides.

"We need ways to do less," Andy said, "and we need community decisions to decide what we are going to do."

---

[2] Andrew L. Jameton, "Chapter 14B: Paediatric Nursing Ethics," in *Ethics and Perinatology*, ed. Goldworth, Silverman, Stevenson, and Young, 427–443. New York: Oxford University Press, 1995.

Chapter 17

Sharing Responsibility

Will communities make rational decisions? Will they accept the enormous challenges they face? Can communities learn how to do less in some areas and more in others with an eye to achieving social justice and ensuring basic human rights for more of their members?

Millions of families—and "millions" is an accurate figure—need help right now coping with the daunting problems of providing meaningful lives for their incompletely rescued children.

Acknowledging their existence is the first step.

Inclusion is the second.

Providing them with help proactively is the third.

Communities, institutions, governments, and individuals can all do something. Those who continue to marginalize and ignore families who are dealing with the enormous morbidity associated with caring for sick children are, as the cliché expresses it, part of the problem.

Many social, political, and economic structures that have failed to provide support for families need to be fixed.

So do regulations, services, and structures that failed to shield children from harms when they were born or inflicted harms directly on them. (I refer here to Baby Doe and BAIPA regulations, prenatal education, and some

NICU practices and procedures. As Siva once put it, "Use of medical and technological advances might help to save more lives but we must also pay attention to whether these advances also decrease morbidity over time.") Until these are fixed, children born in the future remain in jeopardy.

TRIVIAL PURSUITS

The entire baby-making enterprise needs closer scrutiny. We should stop endorsing technologies and practices that enable people to mastermind pregnancies for foolish reasons and that have the potential to hurt babies. Three obvious ones are these: elective early deliveries of babies merely to avoid the inconvenience of waiting for the pregnancy to end, spinning and separating sperm in centrifuges specifically to engineer girl babies or boys, and condoning pregnancies in women who are in their late forties, fifties, and sixties.

One would be hard pressed to show how anyone is truly thinking about the well-being of the future baby with any of these interventions. We have, for example, no way to know what all of the physical and chemical changes are in the last days or minutes of a pregnancy that might be absolutely crucial for the future healthy development of the individual. Similarly, we have no idea what physical and chemical factors inside the uterus influence embryonic development during the first minutes, hours, and days of conception and implantation. To assume that these important transitional periods can be eliminated without consequences to the child is naïve. To assume that time spent in a test tube equals time spent *in vivo* is simply wrong. And although the desire to be a parent may be as intense in an older woman as it is in a younger one, how fair is it to a child to have a mother who will celebrate her seventieth birthday when that child is celebrating her fourth? (Such a pregnancy was engineered in 2005, and a similar one had been achieved in 2003.)

Nature has not succeeded in 160,000 years (the time since we parted ancestral company from the apes) to perfect childbirth and to get things right in producing a healthy baby every time. And yet humans, smitten with the technological imperative and filled with hubris, continue to believe that they can one-up nature, to the detriment of babies.

RISKY BUSINESS

When a reproductive, genetic, or rescue technology makes sense, it still should be embraced with appropriate caution. Technologies, like nature, are fallible.

One mother I interviewed, for example, had been unable to conceive for many years. She went to a fertility specialist, who implanted three embryos in her uterus. Somewhere along the way, one of the embryos split in half. Her quadruplets—healthy identical twin girls, a healthy boy, and a boy with Down syndrome—were two years old when she gave birth to another healthy baby boy, conceived naturally and unexpectedly.

Other women, who also are unable to conceive easily but are not able to afford the high-priced route of in vitro fertilization and implantation, try an even riskier intervention—fertility drugs. These drugs are the ones that lead to the births of the highest multiples—quintuplets, sextuplets, septuplets.

Higher-multiple pregnancies have become less frequent in recent years, in part because obstetricians finally accepted their responsibilities to monitor ovulation more closely and to caution women under their care against becoming pregnant in months when too many eggs had been released. But in the years that passed before this self-regulation came about, many higher-multiple pregnancies occurred, and many of the children today are living with profound disabilities.

SOLIDARITY

I have always been a lover of babies. As a child—the baby of the family—I played constantly with dolls and with babies who lived in the neighborhood.

I was fortunate to give birth to a healthy baby girl at full term on July 12, 1977. The pediatrician walked into my room after she examined my baby and said, "Your baby is perfect."

Her exquisite word choice thrilled me then and has remained emblazoned on my brain. Those words surely are the ones that all new parents would want to hear. (I also noticed and was proud that she had written A+ on my baby's incubator, but that turned out to be my daughter's blood type.)

I was fortunate again on August 28, 1980, to give birth to another perfect, healthy baby girl at full term.

I was not fooled or complacent, though, thinking that all births are straightforward, as those two had been. I had experienced a very painful miscarriage one year before my first daughter was born. I knew intense sadness at losing a wanted pregnancy, and I felt intense yearning to have a child, which I had not been immediately able to do.

The six years that I spent visiting NICUs and talking to parents and neonatal intensivists immersed me in the world of babies whose lives did not start easily, as did my daughters' lives. The world of at-risk babies was a world that I, like so many others, had known very little about.

I have learned that babies matter, but so do their families and the communities in which they live.

Now that I have seen so many struggling babies and their families, I neither can nor want to turn my back on them.

Bibliography

Carter, Brian S. and Marcia Levetown, *Palliative Care for Infants, Children, and Adolescents*, New York: Johns Hopkins University Press, 2004.

Catlin, Anita and Brian Carter, "Creation of a Neonatal End-of-Life Palliative Care Protocol," *Journal of Perinatolgy*, 2002, 22(3): 184–195.

Catlin, Anita, "Thinking Outside the Box: Prenatal Care and the Call for a Prenatal Advance Directive," *Journal of Perinatal and Neonatal Nursing*, 2005, 19(2): 169–176.

Charlie Foundation. http://www.charliefoundation.org/

Chromosome Deletion Outreach, Inc. http://www.chromodisorder.org/

Crane, Sam, *Aidan's Way: The Story of a Boy's Life and a Father's Journey*, Naperville, IL: Source Books, Inc., 2003.

Culver, Gloria et al, letter to the editor, "Informed Decisions for Extremely Low-Birth-Weight Infants," *Journal of the American Medical Association*, 2000, 283(24): 3201.

Finer, Neil et al, "Postnatal Steroids: Short-term Gain, Long-term Pain?" *Journal of Pediatrics*, 2000, 137(1): 9–13.

Frohock, Fred M., *Special Care*, Chicago: University of Chicago Press, 1986.

Ginsberg, Debra, *Raising Blaze: Bringing Up an Extraordinary Son in an Ordinary World*, New York: Perennial, 2002.

Harrison, Helen, letter to the editor, *Journal of Perinatology*, 2001, 15(6): 522.

Harrison, Helen, "Making Lemonade: A Parent's View of 'Quality of Life' Studies," *Journal of Clinical Ethics*, 2001, 12(3): 239–250.

Harrison, Helen, *The Premature Baby Book*, New York: St. Martin's Griffin, 1983.

Harrison, Helen, "The Principles for Family-Centered Neonatal Care," *Pediatrics*, 1993, 92(5): 643–650.

Hippocratic Oath—Modern Version. http://www.pbs.org/wgbh/nova/doctors/oath_modern.html

Jameton, Andrew L., "Chapter 14B: Paediatric Nursing Ethics," in *Ethics and Perinatology*, ed. Goldworth, Silverman, Stevenson, and Young, 427–443. New York: Oxford University Press, 1995.

Kopelman, Loretta M., "Are the 21-Year-Old Baby Doe Rules Misunderstood or Mistaken?" *Pediatrics*, 2005, 115: 797–802.

Kopelman, Loretta M., Thomas G. Irons, Arthur E. Kopelman, "Neonatologists Judge the 'Baby Doe' Regulations," *New England Journal of Medicine*, 1988, 318(11): 677–683.

Kuebelbeck, Amy, *Waiting for Gabriel*, Chicago: Loyola Press, 2003.

Kupfer, Fern, *Before and After Zachariah*, Chicago: Academy Chicago Publishers, 1988.

Kuusisto, Stephen, *Planet of the Blind*, New York: Delta, 1998.

Lantos, John D. "The Difficulty of Being Anti-NICU," *Literature and Medicine*, 1999, 18(2): 237–240.

Lantos, John D., "Hooked on Neonatology," *Health Affairs*, 2001, 20(5): 233–240.

Lantos, John D., "Pediatric Research: What Is Broken and What Needs to Be Fixed," *Journal of Pediatrics*, 2004, 144: 147–149.

Lawrence, Raymond, "David the 'Bubble Boy' and the Boundaries of the Human," *Journal of the American Medical Association*, 1985, 253(1): 74–76.

Leuthner, Stephen and Robin Pierucci, "Experience with Neonatal Palliative Care Consultation at the Medical College of Wisconsin–Children's Hospital of Wisconsin," *Journal of Palliative Medicine*, 2001, 4(1): 39–46.

Levene, Malcolm, "Is Intensive Care for Very Immature Babies Justified?" *Acta Paediatrica*, 2004, 93:149–152.

Loizeaux, William, *Anna: A Daughter's Life*, New York: Arcade Publishing, 1993.

Michael's website: A preemie's journey from early birth to special needs. www.michaelrigaud.co.uk

Moreno, Jonathan D., *Is There an Ethicist in the House? On the Cutting Edge of Bioethics*, Bloomington and Indianapolis: Indiana University Press, 2005.

Neonatology and the Rights of Families. http://www.narof.org/

Oe, Kenzaburo, *A Personal Matter*, New York: Grove Press, 1969.

Paris, John J. and Frank Reardon, "Bad Cases Make Bad Law: HCA v. Miller Is Not a Guide for Resuscitation of Extremely Premature Newborns," *Journal of Perinatology*, 2001, 21: 541–544.

Pediatrics Medical Group. http://www.pediatrix.com/

Pence, Gregory, *Classic Cases in Medical Ethics*, New York: McGraw-Hill, 4th ed., 2004.

Pierce, Jessica and Andrew Jameton, *The Ethics of Environmentally Responsible Health Care*, New York: Oxford University Press, 2004.

Postman, Neil, *Technopoly: The Surrender of Culture to Technology*, New York: Vintage Books, 1993.

ProactiveParents. http://www.proactiveparents.co.nz/about.htm

Rogoff, Marianne, *Sylvie's Life*, Berkeley, CA: Zenobia Press, 1995.

Rothman, Barbara Katz, *The Book of Life*, New York: Beacon Press, 2001.

Rothman, Barbara Katz, *The Tentative Pregnancy*, New York: W. W. Norton and Co., 1993.

Sayeed, Sadath A., "Baby Doe Redux? The Department of Health and Human Services and the Born-Alive Infants Protection Act of 2002: A Cautionary Note on the Normative Neonatal Practice," *Pediatrics*, 2005, 116(4): 576–585.

Silverman, William A., "Incubator-Baby Side Shows," *Pediatrics*, 1979, 64(2): 127–141.

Silverman, William A., "Mandatory Rescue of Fetal Infants," *Paediatric and Perinatal Epidemiology*, 2005, 19(2): 86–87.

Silverman, William A., "Overtreatment of Neonates? A Personal Retrospective," *Pediatrics*, 1992, 90(6): 971–976.

Silverman, William A., *Retrolental Fibroplasia: A Modern Parable (Monographs in Neonatology)*, New York: Grune & Stratton, Inc., 1980.

Silverman, William A., *Where's the Evidence?* New York: Oxford University Press, 1998.

Stimpson, Jeff, *Alex: The Fathering of a Preemie*, Chicago: Academy Chicago Publishers, 2004.

Unique but not alone. Rare chromosome support group. http://www.rare chromo.org/html/home.asp

Veatch, Robert, *The Basics of Bioethics*, Upper Saddle River, NJ: Prentice Hall, 2000.

Veatch, Robert, *Disrupted Dialogue: Medical Ethics and the Collapse of Physician-Humanist Communication*, USA: Oxford University Press, 2004.

Veatch, Robert, *Medical Ethics*, Boston, MA: Jones and Bartlett, 1997.

About the Author

Ruth Levy Guyer is a respected science and medical writer. She teaches courses in bioethics, infectious disease, and social justice at Haverford College and is a regular commentator on National Public Radio's weekend *All Things Considered*. She has written about birth, pregnancy, new reproductive technologies, cloning, genetic engineering, and other medical and scientific subjects that have ethical implications. Her work has been published in the *American Journal of Bioethics, Bioethics Forum, Science Magazine*, the *American Journal of Public Health*, the *Washington Post*, the *St. Louis Post Dispatch*, and elsewhere. She has taught writing courses at Johns Hopkins University, Carleton College, UCLA Medical School, the National Institutes of Health, and the independent Bethesda Writer's Center. Her PhD is in immunology. She lives in Bethesda, MD.

Index